UNDERSTANDING TYPE 2 DIABETES

SIMPLE STEPS TO AVOID COMPLICATIONS, REDUCE MEDICAL EXPENSES, DECREASE STRESS, AND LIVE A HEALTHY & PROACTIVE LIFE

DR. ASHLEY SULLIVAN, PHARMD, RPH, MBA

Copyright © 2023 Dr. Ashley Sullivan, PharmD, RPh, MBA. All rights reserved.

The content within this book may not be reproduced, duplicated, or transmitted without direct written permission from the author or the publisher.

Under no circumstances will any blame or legal responsibility be held against the publisher, or author, for any damages, reparation, or monetary loss due to the information contained within this book, either directly or indirectly.

Legal Notice:

This book is copyright protected. It is only for personal use. You cannot amend, distribute, sell, use, quote, or paraphrase any part of the content within this book, without the consent of the author or publisher.

Disclaimer Notice:

Please note the information contained within this document is for educational and entertainment purposes only. All effort has been expended to present accurate, up-to-date, reliable, and complete information. No warranties of any kind are declared or implied. Readers acknowledge that the author is not engaged in the rendering of legal, financial, medical, or professional advice. The content within this book has been derived from various sources. Please consult a licensed professional before attempting any techniques outlined in this book.

By reading this document, the reader agrees that under no circumstances is the author responsible for any losses, direct or indirect, that are incurred as a result of the use of the information contained within this document, including, but not limited to, errors, omissions, or inaccuracies.

CONTENTS

Introduction	7
1. WHAT IS TYPE 2 DIABETES?	13
What is Type 2 Diabetes?	13
Why Are So Many People Affected?	16
The History Behind Type 2 Diabetes	19
What Are the Risk Factors for Diabetes?	23
What Are the Most Common Diabetes Symptoms?	25
What Are Some Other Signs That You Might Have Type 2 Diabetes?	27
What is the Difference Between Type 1 and Type 2 Diabetes?	28
How is Diabetes Diagnosed?	30
2. UNDERSTANDING INSULIN AND BLOOD SUGAR	33
What Role Does Insulin Play in the Body?	34
What is Blood Glucose?	36
What Role Does the Pancreas Play?	37
How Does Glucose Metabolism Work?	38
What Makes Your Glucose Metabolism Get Out of Whack?	39
Carbs and Diabetes	41
How Insulin Resistance Occurs	47
The Impact of High Blood Sugar on the Body	48
The Relationship Between Insulin and Blood Sugar	50
3. THE CAUSES AND PREVENTION OF DIABETES	53
What Genetic Factors Contribute to Diabetes?	54
Which Lifestyle Choices Impact Diabetes Risk?	56

Other Risk Factors for Diabetes 58
The Role of Sleep and Stress in Diabetes Prevention 61
Steroid Use and Diabetes 62

4. TREATMENT OPTIONS FOR DIABETES 67
Lifestyle Changes as a First-Line Treatment 68
Medication for Blood Sugar Control 69
The Importance of Insulin Therapy 73
How, When, and Why - Monitoring Blood Sugar Levels 75
The Importance of Regular Medical Check-ups 84

5. MANAGING DIABETES THROUGH DIET 87
The Role of Carbohydrates, Fats, and Proteins in Blood Sugar Control 88
Recommended Dietary Guidelines 90
What About Dietary Supplements? 92
Guidance on Creating Your Own Healthy Eating Plan 94
Putting Together a Basic Menu Plan 99
How to Read and Understand Food Labels 102
Smoking and Diabetes 105
Sleep and Diabetes 107
Stress and Diabetes 109

6. EXERCISE AND PHYSICAL ACTIVITY FOR DIABETES MANAGEMENT 115
Why You Need to Get Active and Start Exercising 117
Diabetes and Exercise: When to Monitor Your Blood Sugar 119
Different Types of Exercise and How They Affect Blood Sugar 120
Safety Considerations for Exercise With Diabetes 122
Importance of Incorporating Physical Activity into Your Daily Life 123

7. MANAGING TYPE 2 DIABETES
   COMPLICATIONS   125
   What Are the Risks of Uncontrolled Glucose
   Complications?   126

8. THE ROLE OF MEDICATIONS IN TYPE 2
   DIABETES MANAGEMENT   137
   Types of Medications for Blood Sugar Control   138
   Which Other Medications Can Interfere With
   Diabetes Medications?   146
   Benefits and Risks of Medication Therapy   150
   What to Do if Your Diabetes Medication Isn't
   Working   151
   Lifestyle Changes vs Medication: Which is
   Best?   151
   The Cost of Insulin   152
   Why It's So Important to Stick to Your
   Medication Schedule   153

9. MENTAL HEALTH AND EMOTIONAL
   WELL-BEING WITH DIABETES   155
   Emotional Impact of a Diabetes Diagnosis   156
   Strategies for Coping with the Emotional and
   Psychological Challenges of Diabetes   158
   Importance of Seeking Support   159
   The Role of Stress and Anxiety in Blood Sugar
   Control   162
   How to Prioritize Self-Care and Mental Health
   in Diabetes Management   163

10. ADVOCATING FOR YOUR HEALTH WITH
    TYPE 2 DIABETES   167
    Why it's Important to Be an Active Participant
    in Healthcare Decisions   168
    What to Consider When Communicating with
    Healthcare Professionals   169
    Patient Rights as a Diabetic   172
    The Role of Technology in Diabetes
    Management   173

Self-Advocacy for Better Health Outcomes 175
Special Considerations for Diabetes
Management 177

Conclusion 181
Glossary 185
References 189

INTRODUCTION

According to the Centers for Disease Control and Prevention (CDC), over 34 million Americans have diabetes. 90 to 95% of those cases are type 2 diabetes.

Whether you've recently been diagnosed with type 2 diabetes or you've been living with it for many years, keeping your blood sugar under control can be an overwhelming, lonely experience.

I say this as someone who has worked in the medical field for many years. I have seen firsthand the frustration my patients have when they go to the pharmacy to pick up insulin or testing supplies and they have high costs even with insurance. I have seen the fear in their eyes when they've been told that they're at risk for vision problems or kidney disease. I sense the anxiety they're feeling, and my heart goes out to everyone who has been affected by this disease.

But know this - you are not alone.

Diabetes is incredibly common, as you can see from the statistic above, but it's also important to note that you are *not* just a statistic. You are a person. And I see you.

As someone with diabetes, you may be faced with a laundry list of symptoms and potential complications. Your gut instinct might be to turn to your doctor for advice, but the reality is that not all of us have doctors whom we feel like we can confide in. There are so many barriers to receiving proper treatment, and it is tough to know what steps to take.

If you or someone you love has recently been diagnosed with type 2 diabetes, it is understandable that you may feel overwhelmed and unsure of where to start. Type 2 diabetes is a chronic condition that affects millions of people worldwide and managing it can be challenging.

As you already know, type 2 diabetes is a condition where the body either does not produce enough insulin or is not able to use insulin effectively. Insulin is a hormone that is responsible for regulating blood sugar levels in the body.

Common symptoms of type 2 diabetes include frequent urination, excessive thirst, fatigue, and blurred vision. Understanding these symptoms and how they relate to the condition can help you manage it better, but as someone who has the disease, you might not fully understand how these specific symptoms will affect you specifically - after all, everybody is different.

One of the biggest challenges of managing type 2 diabetes is controlling blood sugar levels, which can fluctuate based on numerous factors such as diet, exercise, stress, and medication.

Monitoring your blood sugar levels regularly can provide insight into how these factors affect your body, but again, it is a tough balance to strike between proper nutrition, exercise, stress, and medication. Often, the recommendations given to us by medical professionals are generalized - they are not customized to your unique situation.

Sure, you should be limiting stress in your day-to-day life. But you are the parent of three kids under five years old, you have a demanding 40-hour-a-week job, and various life stressors on top of that - stressors you cannot necessarily avoid. You need advice that is tailored to your unique situation.

To make matters worse, there are many stressful factors that complicate this disease. We know that people with type 2 diabetes are at risk for a range of complications, including nerve damage, vision problems, kidney disease, and heart disease. But there is a good chance you don't want to live in constant fear of those progressive symptoms.

The cost of managing type 2 diabetes can be high, including regular doctor visits, medications, and medical devices such as glucose meters and insulin pumps. Even if you have excellent insurance, it is tough to predict what will and won't be covered.

It is safe to say that receiving a diagnosis of type 2 diabetes can be emotionally challenging - and it can impact your mental health and self-esteem.

The fear of these complications and potential expenses can be overwhelming and cause anxiety, but it is important to remember that with proper management, these risks can be significantly reduced. Regular check-ups with your doctor and taking medications as prescribed can help prevent complications from worsening. Having the right information and a basic knowledge of what you are up against is also helpful.

That is where I come in.

Managing type 2 diabetes can be a lonely experience, and you could benefit from emotional and social support to help you stay motivated and positive. I want to help alleviate some of your emotional burden by teaching you everything you need to know about how to manage your diabetes so you can live a fulfilling, happy, and stress-free life (or at least, somewhat stress-free!) life.

I know that a diagnosis of type 2 diabetes comes with a lot of *really* big feelings. You might be angry that others misunderstand your condition or angry at presumptions that your diabetes was caused by poor lifestyle decisions you made.

You might feel frustrated or helpless, upset that your symptoms are interfering with your daily life. You might be unsure of how you are going to afford next month's medications or doctors' appointments. You might feel judged or criticized by others. You might feel like you are just going through the motions, trying to get from one day to the next, rather than being able to enjoy life.

Again. You are not alone. These feelings are normal, and I want to help you work through them.

Proper education is the first step in any journey, and that is where this book comes in. If you want to have the confidence you need to manage your diabetes, you need to understand everything there is to know about it. You need to understand the best recommendations for:

- Stress management
- Nutrition and exercise
- Lifestyle adjustments and essential diet control tips as a first line of defense to manage your condition
- Managing your blood sugar levels
- Medication treatment options

I'll give you a complete review of the technology, trends, and modern science around the condition - no more outdated pamphlets from the waiting room of your doctor's office.

And most importantly, I'll give you the knowledge and empowerment you need to advocate for yourself - and for a person-centered approach to managing your condition. There is a glossary of medical terms at the end of the book before the references. Citations follow the end of the book, although a lot of the information presented is from my professional education and work experience.

Whether your goal is to be able to manage your symptoms without medication or just to reduce your symptoms, this book is for you.

I did not come by this knowledge overnight. As I mentioned earlier, I have worked for several years in the medical field, and I've worked closely with dozens of patients just like you. I know where you are coming from. I know how hard this is. And I want to help you better understand diabetes.

Are you ready to get started? Let us take a deep dive into type 2 diabetes - and let's get you on the track toward a brighter, more empowered future.

1

WHAT IS TYPE 2 DIABETES?

Diabetes is a chronic condition that affects millions of people around the world. According to the 2020 National Diabetes Statistics Report, around 34.2 million people in the United States have diabetes, which accounts for 10.5% of the US population. Diabetes is a disease that impacts the way the body processes blood sugar or glucose. Broadly speaking, there are two types of diabetes: type 1 and type 2. This book will dive into type 2 diabetes, but it is important to note that there are many commonalities shared between the two.

WHAT IS TYPE 2 DIABETES?

Type 2 Diabetes is a chronic condition that occurs when your body becomes resistant to insulin, or when the pancreas produces inadequate insulin. Insulin is a hormone that regulates blood sugar, and without it, glucose surges in your bloodstream and can cause serious problems.

Over time, high levels of glucose in the blood can lead to severe complications such as neuropathy (nerve pain), blindness, and kidney problems. Type 2 Diabetes is the most diagnosed type of diabetes, with nearly 90% of the diabetes cases being Type 2 in the US.

What Causes Type 2 Diabetes?

Type 2 diabetes is caused by a combination of genetic and environmental factors. Individuals with a family history of the disease are more likely to develop it.

Obesity, a sedentary lifestyle, and poor dietary habits also increase the risk of developing type 2 diabetes. People with metabolic syndrome, a condition that includes high blood pressure and elevated cholesterol levels, are also at risk of developing type 2 diabetes.

Regardless of the cause, type 2 diabetes occurs when the body becomes resistant to insulin or when the pancreas fails to produce enough insulin, a hormone that regulates blood sugar levels.

Is Type 2 Diabetes Serious?

You probably already know this, but diabetes can be serious if left untreated. High levels of glucose in the blood can cause damage to various organs and lead to complications such as blindness, kidney disease, nerve damage, heart disease, and stroke.

Can Type 2 Diabetes Be Cured?

While type 2 diabetes cannot be cured, it can be managed with proper treatment and lifestyle changes. The goal of treatment is to keep blood sugar levels in the target range to prevent complications.

Treatment may involve medications such as metformin, controlling blood pressure and cholesterol levels, and regular exercise and weight loss. In some cases, bariatric surgery may be considered if obesity is an underlying issue related to the diagnosis of diabetes.

Many people can reduce their medications if they make lifestyle changes to help control their blood glucose levels. You should always work with your medical provider when making changes and communicate your goals for treatment.

Type 2 Diabetes Treatment Options

The treatment for type 2 diabetes may vary depending on an individual's unique needs. The treatment plan may include medications that help lower blood sugar levels and improve insulin sensitivity, such as metformin, sulfonylureas (glipizide, glimepiride, glyburide), or thiazolidinediones (pioglitazone). These options are discussed further into the book.

Perhaps more importantly, lifestyle changes such as weight loss, regular exercise, and healthy eating can help manage blood sugar, blood pressure, and cholesterol.

It is essential to work closely with a healthcare provider to develop a personalized treatment plan that works best for you. In this book, I will walk you through some potential treatment options that you may find effective and helpful.

WHY ARE SO MANY PEOPLE AFFECTED?

In the United States alone, more than 34 million people have diabetes, and millions of others are at risk of developing the disease. Type 2 diabetes is on the rise, and several factors contribute to this alarming trend.

Obesity

The first and most significant factor contributing to the rise in type 2 diabetes is obesity.

In the US, obesity has been on the increase over the past 15 years, and there has been an increase in diabetes rates to correspond with that rise. There are a few reasons for this, but the most significant to note is that obesity increases insulin resistance, which leads to high levels of glucose in the blood, leading to diabetes.

Lack of Physical Activity

Lack of physical activity is another contributing factor to the rise in type 2 diabetes. Our lifestyle has become increasingly sedentary, with a lot of time spent in front of screens. This means that exercise is not prioritized, and this lack of physical activity leads to weight gain and other health problems, including diabetes.

There is one story I'd like to mention here to illustrate the huge impact that physical activity has on diabetes. One man, Roger Hare, was diagnosed with type-2 diabetes in 2019. He told his story to a WebMD reporter shortly after his diagnosis. Like most people, he faced a variety of emotions upon hearing that he had diabetes. He was angry, panicked, and confused. He thought the world was coming to an end. However, he acted quickly, putting a plan together to drop some weight.

Although medication and nutrition played a big part in his weight loss (and reduction in diabetes symptoms), Hare noted the extreme importance of being active, stating, "Exercise plays a big role. I go to the gym two or three times a week for cardio and strength training. I normally start with 15-20 minutes on the treadmill. Then I will do some weightlifting and floor exercises. I cool down with another 10-15 minutes on the treadmill."

While it has not always been easy, he lost 40 pounds and dropped his A1C by more than 6 points. That is remarkable!

Dietary Changes

Dietary changes are also responsible for the increase in type 2 diabetes.

We are far more likely to eat foods that are high in sugar (even those that are not necessarily desserts - did you know that store-bought tomato sauce has a whopping 10 grams of sugar?). Carbonated drinks, packaged ready-to-eat foods, and fried foods, are all common factors leading to chronic inflammation and diabetes as well.

Awareness & Changes in Diagnostic Criteria

Awareness also plays a role in the rise of type 2 diabetes. There has been an increase in awareness regarding the health effects of diabetes and the importance of regular check-ups.

People are getting evaluated for diabetes earlier. That is a good thing, since it means that early detection is being prioritized and that people are taking the necessary measures to prevent the disease, but it also results in higher rates of diabetes being reported.

Doctors are now able to recommend exercises and dietary changes not just for people who have diabetes, but also those with prediabetes, which is the stage in which blood sugar levels are elevated, but not at the level of "full-blown" diabetes. There are about 96 million people in the US (aged

18 years or older) who have prediabetes. This is estimated to be around 38% of the population.

There are new tests available for diabetes as well. A new blood test, HbA1C, makes it possible to diagnose diabetes without the need for fasting for 12 hours. It is much more reliable and effective at diagnosing diabetes early on, especially in younger people.

Aging Population

Finally, the aging population is a contributing factor to the rise in type 2 diabetes. As we age, our body's ability to use insulin decreases, increasing the risk of developing diabetes.

With the baby-boomer generation reaching retirement age, there has been a corresponding (and expected) surge in diabetes cases among older adults.

THE HISTORY BEHIND TYPE 2 DIABETES

Now that you know what diabetes is and why it has become more common, let's take a closer look at the history behind the disease. Understanding our history is the best way to make smart, informed decisions in the future.

Believe it or not, the history of diabetes dates back to ancient times when it was described by physicians as a mysterious disease that caused frequent urination and emaciation (thin and weak).

The first recorded symptoms of diabetes were documented in 1552 B.C. by Hesy-Ra, an Egyptian physician who observed excessive urination as a key symptom of this befuddling disease that caused emaciation.

However, it was not until centuries later that physicians started to gain a better understanding of this condition. In 150 AD, the Greek doctor Arateus described diabetes as "the melting down of flesh and limbs into urine," thus highlighting the connection between sugar in urine and diabetes.

During the Middle Ages, a group of people began to diagnose diabetes. The way they did this was not with any fancy diagnostic test, but simply by tasting the urine of people who were believed to have diabetes. If the urine tasted sweet, the patient was diagnosed with diabetes. This group of people was known as "water tasters," and this is how diabetes was diagnosed for many centuries.

In 1675, the word "mellitus," which translates to honey, was added to the name "diabetes," which itself translated to the word "siphon." This was done to acknowledge the sweet, honey-like taste of the patient's urine. Believe it or not, it wasn't until later, in the 1800s, that scientists invented chemical tests to detect the presence of sugar in urine, making the diagnosis process much simpler (and not so unappetizing).

However, it was even earlier than that when physicians discovered that dietary changes could help manage diabetes.

They recommended that their patients eat only the fat and meat of animals or consume substantial amounts of sugar. Now we know how damaging sugar is to our body and how much it contributes to the development of diabetes, but back then they did not understand diabetes.

During the Franco-Prussian War of the early 1870s, a French physician Apollinaire Bouchardat noted that the symptoms of his diabetic patients showed a dramatic improvement. This was due to the cause of food rationing related to the war. As a result, Bouchardat created individualized diets that served as a core component of diabetes treatments.

In the early 1900s, fad diets became popular as treatments for diabetes. The "oat cure," "potato therapy," and the "starvation diet" were the most famous diets of the time. The oat cure involved consuming substantial amounts of oatmeal, while the potato therapy revolved around eating only potatoes for several days.

The starvation diet, on the other hand, involved severely restricting calories to induce weight loss. While these diets may have helped some diabetes patients temporarily, they were not sustainable and often did more harm than good.

In 1916, Boston scientist Elliott Joslin published *The Treatment of Diabetes Mellitus*, a textbook that established him as one of the world's leading diabetes experts. In his book, Joslin said that a fasting diet, when combined with physical activity, could reduce the mortality risk for diabetes patients.

This was a significant milestone in the development of diabetes management and the way we treat diabetes today.

Despite all these advances and research, before the discovery of insulin, diabetes almost always resulted in premature death. Insulin was discovered and first used in 1889 when Oskar Minkowski and Joseph von Mering found that the removal of a dog's pancreas could synthetically induce diabetes.

Then, in the 1920s, scientists discovered insulin, a hormone produced by the pancreas that is necessary to regulate blood sugar levels. As you might expect, this breakthrough discovery was an absolute game-changer in the treatment of diabetes. People with diabetes, who were once condemned to a life of extreme diets and constant monitoring, could now manage their condition with regular insulin injections.

Today, diabetes is still a major health concern, but of course, it's much more well-understood. People aged 40 and above are at the highest risk. However, recent studies show that young adults ages 18-34 are also at risk. In fact, the number of young adults being diagnosed with diabetes is on the rise. Your risk is higher if you are African Caribbean, Black African, or South Asian - or if you're male.

While it's important to note that while certain age groups and demographics are at a higher risk, diabetes can affect anyone at any age. It is also not an issue that's exclusive to the US. While there are 338 million people with diabetes in the United States as of 2023, there are more than a billion people each in China and India with the disease.

Let me say it again, as if these statistics do not demonstrate it well enough - you're not alone! The good news is that there are more researchers devoted to studying diabetes now, in 2023, than ever before and lots of good things are happening.

WHAT ARE THE RISK FACTORS FOR DIABETES?

Next, you might be wondering what makes you more likely to develop diabetes. While there are always outliers, there are a few common risk factors present in most cases of diagnosed diabetes.

Again, one significant risk factor for diabetes is weight. Being overweight or obese is a primary risk factor for developing type 2 diabetes. The more excess body fat you carry, particularly around your waistline, the more likely you are to develop diabetes.

It is so important to maintain a healthy weight to reduce your risk of developing diabetes. Regular exercise and a healthy diet can help you achieve this.

Another crucial factor to consider is inactivity. Living a sedentary lifestyle can increase your risk of developing diabetes, irrespective of your weight. Physical activity can help control your weight, improve glucose utilization, and increase your cells' insulin sensitivity.

Therefore, finding ways to get active, whether through exercise, walking, or other physical activities (or a combination, like our story of Roger Hare from above), can help reduce your risk of developing diabetes.

Family history is another significant factor to consider. People who have immediate family members with type 2 diabetes are at a higher risk of developing the condition. Therefore, regularly checking your blood sugar levels and having a conversation with your doctor about your family history can help diagnose and manage the condition early.

Other risk factors include age, cholesterol levels, prediabetes, and pregnancy-related risks. As you age, your risk for developing diabetes increases, particularly if you are over 35 years old.

Low levels of high-density lipoprotein (HDL), or "good" cholesterol, and elevated levels of triglycerides can also increase your risk of diabetes. Having prediabetes or a previous history of gestational diabetes or giving birth to a baby weighing more than nine pounds can also make you more susceptible to diabetes as well.

This is a risk factor that is seldom talked about - childbirth. In fact, one story of a diabetes patient, Jenn, as reported to The Johns Hopkins Patient Guide to Diabetes, highlights this well. Jenn was diagnosed with gestational diabetes for each one of her three pregnancies (usually in the third trimester). Even though Jenn is still at risk of developing adult onset type 2 diabetes was able to manage her condition by diet alone while she was pregnant, and it went away after she delivered each of her babies.

Smoking is also a risk factor of diabetes. People who smoke cigarettes are 30% - 40% more likely to develop type 2 diabetes than people who do not smoke. Nicotine can contribute to cells having a decreased response to insulin, resulting in elevated levels of glucose in the blood.

WHAT ARE THE MOST COMMON DIABETES SYMPTOMS?

One of the key aspects of managing type 2 diabetes is being aware of the symptoms. You may have some or all of these, but knowing about each of them is key to managing the condition successfully.

- **Increased thirst:** Do you feel like you are always reaching for a drink? Excessive thirst is one of the most common symptoms of diabetes. When your blood sugar levels rise, your body tries to get rid of the excess sugar by flushing it out through urine, but this can leave you dehydrated.
- **Frequent urination:** If you are suddenly finding yourself making more trips to the bathroom than usual, it could be another sign of diabetes. High

blood sugar levels can cause your kidneys to work overtime, trying to filter out the excess sugar. This can lead to more frequent trips to the bathroom, especially at night.

- **Increased hunger:** Constant hunger, even after eating, is another common symptom of diabetes. When your body cannot get the glucose it needs from food, it goes into overdrive looking for more fuel, which can result in increased hunger and food cravings.
- **Unintended weight loss**: Losing weight without trying might sound like a dream for some, but when it happens suddenly and without explanation, it can be a cause for concern (especially if you have that elevated appetite we mentioned earlier). In some people with diabetes, the body may start burning fat and muscle for energy instead of glucose, leading to unintentional weight loss.
- **Fatigue**: Diabetes can make you feel more fatigued than usual, because your body can't extract enough glucose from the food you eat for energy. This can leave you feeling depleted and sluggish, even after a good night's sleep.

WHAT ARE SOME OTHER SIGNS THAT YOU MIGHT HAVE TYPE 2 DIABETES?

If you have type 2 diabetes, you have a higher risk of suffering from various other health problems. Sometimes, it is these secondary issues that lead people to seek medical attention for their diabetes rather than the symptoms listed above.

For instance, nerve damage is one common complication that many people with Type 2 diabetes encounter. If you have high blood sugar levels for an extended period, your nerves can get damaged or even destroyed, leading to a condition called neuropathy. This can cause you to feel numbness, tingling, or loss of sensation in your limbs.

People with diabetes can also develop a condition known as autonomic neuropathy. This happens when the nerves controlling the heart and blood vessels get damaged or destroyed. Consequently, it may be harder to control your blood pressure, heartbeat, and digestion.

High blood sugar levels damage the blood vessels and lead to inflammation in the kidneys, which can eventually cause kidney disease. People with Type 2 diabetes are also 2-4 times more likely to develop eye-related complications than those without it.

Moreover, people with diabetes may also experience sleep apnea, a condition characterized by the cessation of breathing for short periods during sleep. Obesity is the primary contributing factor behind both Type 2 diabetes and sleep apnea.

Another less-known symptom of Type 2 diabetes is dementia. People with uncontrolled blood sugar levels are at a higher risk of developing Alzheimer's disease or other related disorders. In some studies, it has been found that poor control of blood sugar is linked to a more rapid decline in memory and other cognitive functions.

Finally, Type 2 diabetes can affect your skin in various ways. We may notice yellow, reddish, or brown patches on our skin, and around the eyes, they may occur in clusters that look like pimples. You may notice the appearance of velvety, dark areas on your skin. You may also experience skin infections, open sores, shin spots, red-yellow bumps, dryness, itchiness, and skin tags.

WHAT IS THE DIFFERENCE BETWEEN TYPE 1 AND TYPE 2 DIABETES?

These two types of diabetes are commonly grouped together, but they are very different. In fact, they have a different impact on your health, diagnosis, and treatment.

So, what is the main difference between type 1 and type 2 diabetes? Type 1 diabetes is an autoimmune disease where your immune system attacks and destroys the cells in your pancreas that make insulin. Insulin is a hormone that allows your body to use sugar for energy.

Without insulin, sugar builds up in your bloodstream and can lead to serious health problems. Type 1 diabetes typically develops in childhood or young adulthood and requires lifelong insulin therapy.

On the other hand, type 2 diabetes is a metabolic disorder where your body either doesn't produce enough insulin or can't use insulin effectively. This is known as insulin resistance.

Unlike type 1 diabetes, type 2 diabetes can be prevented or delayed with lifestyle changes like a healthy diet and regular exercise. However, if left untreated, it can lead to serious health complications.

Type 1 diabetes affects only 8% of people with diabetes, while type 2 diabetes accounts for about 90% of cases, as I mentioned earlier. However, the signs and symptoms of both types of diabetes can be similar, such as increased thirst, frequent urination, and blurred vision.

Another difference between type 1 and type 2 diabetes is related to the risk factors. Type 1 diabetes is thought to be caused by a combination of genetic and environmental factors, such as exposure to viruses and other triggers.

Type 2 diabetes, on the other hand, is associated with risk factors like obesity, inactivity, and unhealthy eating habits. If you have a family history of diabetes, you are also at higher risk of developing type 2 diabetes.

Diagnosing the two different types of diabetes is also different - something I'll address in greater detail below.

HOW IS DIABETES DIAGNOSED?

The most common way of diagnosing type 2 diabetes is through the A1C test. This test measures your average blood sugar level over the past two to three months.

If your A1C test results indicate a value of 6.5% or higher on two separate tests, then you have diabetes. However, if you are experiencing certain conditions or if the A1C test is not available, your healthcare provider may use the following tests to diagnose diabetes.

There is also a random blood sugar test where blood sugar values are expressed in milligrams of sugar per deciliter of blood. Regardless of when you last ate, a blood sugar level of 200 mg/dL or higher indicates diabetes if you are also experiencing symptoms like frequent urination and extreme thirst.

Another test that your healthcare provider may use to diagnose diabetes is a fasting blood sugar test. Your healthcare provider takes a blood sample after you have not eaten overnight.

If your fasting blood glucose level measures less than 100 mg/dL, it is considered healthy. If your level is between 100-125 mg/dL, it is diagnosed as prediabetes.

However, if it is 126 mg/dL or higher on two separate tests, you likely have diabetes.

For the oral glucose tolerance test, you'll need to not eat for a certain amount of time and then drink a sugary liquid at your healthcare provider's office. Your glucose level is then tested periodically for two hours. This test is less commonly used than the others, except during pregnancy.

Now that you know the basics about type 2 diabetes, including its symptoms and diagnosis, let's talk a bit more about blood sugar and insulin. After all, these are two of the most important factors to consider (and insulin, the most important element in the treatment of diabetes) when you're coming up with a treatment plan.

Grab a glass of water and a snack, then come back and keep reading. I'll be here waiting for you!

2

UNDERSTANDING INSULIN AND BLOOD SUGAR

"Insulin is not a cure for diabetes; it is a treatment. It enables the diabetic to burn sufficient carbohydrates so that proteins and fats may be added to the diet in sufficient quantities to provide energy for the economic burdens of life."

— FREDERICK BANTING

If you're someone who's struggling with diabetes, chances are you've heard the word 'insulin' thrown around a lot. But what's insulin, and why is it so important when it comes to diabetes management?

When you eat, your digestive system breaks down the food into glucose, which gets absorbed into your bloodstream. However, for glucose to enter your cells and provide energy, it needs insulin. Insulin is a hormone produced by the pancreas that helps regulate blood sugar levels in your body. If you're diabetic, there are problems with this - the body has become resistant to insulin and can't use it effectively.

Let's take a closer look at how insulin and glucose work together.

WHAT ROLE DOES INSULIN PLAY IN THE BODY?

If you're living with diabetes, you've probably heard the word "insulin" more often than you'd like. This hormone, produced by the pancreas, plays a crucial role in regulating your blood sugar levels.

But how?

Insulin is a hormone that helps our bodies convert glucose (a type of sugar) into energy. When we eat carbohydrates, our digestive system breaks them down into glucose, which then enters the bloodstream. This signals the pancreas to release insulin, which acts like a key to unlock the cells in our muscles, liver, and fat tissue, allowing them to absorb glucose from the blood and use it for energy.

Without insulin, our cells would be starved of glucose, and our blood sugar levels would skyrocket, leading to a condition called hyperglycemia. Over time, uncontrolled hyperglycemia can damage our nerves, blood vessels, kidneys, and eyes, causing serious complications like heart disease, blindness, and nerve damage.

For people living with type 1 diabetes, their pancreas cannot produce insulin, so they must take insulin injections or use an insulin pump to regulate their blood sugar levels. For those with type 2 diabetes, their body becomes resistant to the effects of insulin, so they may need to take medication to help their body use insulin more effectively.

Aside from its role in regulating blood sugar, insulin also plays several other important functions in the body. For example, it helps to stimulate the growth and repair of cells, promotes the storage of fat, and inhibits the breakdown of stored glucose and fat. In addition, insulin acts as a signal to the kidneys to reabsorb glucose, aiding in its conservation.

Interestingly, insulin can also affect our hunger and satiety levels. When we eat a meal, our blood sugar levels spike, causing insulin to be released and helping our cells absorb glucose.

But this also causes a drop in our blood sugar levels, which signals the brain to feel hungry and crave more food. However, insulin also triggers the release of hormones that make us feel full, so we don't overeat.

WHAT IS BLOOD GLUCOSE?

Simply put, blood glucose is the sugar that's carried in our blood and provides energy to our cells. It comes from the food we eat and is one of the main things our bodies use for fuel. Sounds important, right?

But for diabetics, keeping blood glucose levels within a healthy range can be a challenge. In type 1 diabetes, the pancreas can't produce insulin, a hormone that helps regulate blood glucose levels. In type 2 diabetes, the body doesn't use insulin as effectively as it should. Both types can lead to high blood glucose levels, which can cause a variety of health complications if left uncontrolled.

So why is it so important to keep blood glucose levels in check? First and foremost, it can help prevent long-term complications like nerve damage, kidney damage, and eye damage. But it can also have an immediate impact on how we feel day-to-day. High blood glucose levels can make us feel tired, thirsty, and generally unwell. On the other hand, low blood glucose levels can lead to shakiness, dizziness, and even unconsciousness.

Managing blood glucose levels as a diabetic can be a full-time job, but there are a variety of tools and strategies that can make it easier. One of the most important is monitoring your levels regularly through blood glucose testing. You may need to do this several times a day, depending on your treatment plan and the advice of your healthcare provider.

Again, I'll have more information on this for you later in this book.

WHAT ROLE DOES THE PANCREAS PLAY?

As a diabetic, you are probably aware that insulin and glucose management are vital to your health. Both factors play a crucial role in keeping your body functioning correctly. However, do you know which organ in your body is responsible for regulating insulin and glucose levels?

Truth be told, the pancreas is somewhat of an unsung hero when it comes to glucose and insulin management.

The pancreas is a small, spongy gland that is located behind your stomach. It is responsible for the secretion of two important hormones, insulin and glucagon, which regulate blood glucose levels in the body. Insulin is produced by beta cells in the pancreas, which plays a critical role in allowing glucose to enter cells and produce energy.

Meanwhile, glucagon is released by alpha cells in the pancreas and raises blood glucose levels when it drops too low.

Most people are familiar with insulin and know that it's essential for managing blood glucose levels. After we eat, our pancreas releases insulin into our bloodstream, which helps cells absorb glucose from food. In a perfect world, our pancreas produces just enough insulin for our body's needs.

Unfortunately, for diabetics, there's an imbalance - either too little insulin or too much. This imbalance can lead to hyperglycemia (high blood sugar) or hypoglycemia (low blood sugar) - both of which can have harmful effects on your body.

When your body is unable to produce enough insulin or becomes resistant to insulin, it can lead to diabetes.

HOW DOES GLUCOSE METABOLISM WORK?

Glucose, a simple sugar, serves as the primary source of fuel for our bodies. After consuming carbohydrates, such as bread and fruit, they are broken down into glucose molecules in the digestive system. This glucose then enters the bloodstream, where it is transported to cells throughout the body.

To enter these cells, glucose requires insulin, a hormone produced by the pancreas. Insulin attaches to the cells' receptors, signaling for them to open and absorb glucose from the bloodstream. Once inside the cells, glucose can be used for energy or stored for later use.

When the body doesn't produce enough insulin or is unable to properly use it, glucose cannot enter the cells efficiently. As a result, glucose builds up in the bloodstream, leading to high blood sugar levels - diabetes.

Beyond diabetes, glucose metabolism also plays a role in other areas of health. For instance, high blood sugar levels can lead to inflammation, which has been linked to a host of health issues, such as heart disease and cancer. Understanding and managing glucose metabolism can help minimize these risks.

WHAT MAKES YOUR GLUCOSE METABOLISM GET OUT OF WHACK?

If you're a diabetic, then you know how finicky your glucose metabolism can be. One minute it's cruising along, and the next, it's as if it's been thrown off its rocker. But what exactly makes this happen? You won't be surprised to hear that many of the factors that cause an imbalance in your glucose metabolism are the same ones discussed as risk factors for diabetes earlier in this book, in the last chapter.

The most obvious culprit behind a dysfunctional glucose metabolism is a poor diet. Unhealthy eating habits, such as consuming excessive amounts of refined sugars, can lead to spikes in blood sugar, which may cause your body to overload on insulin. In turn, this can cause insulin resistance, which impairs your body's ability to control blood sugar levels effectively.

Regular exercise is essential in maintaining optimal glucose metabolism. Exercise increases your insulin sensitivity, allowing your body to use insulin more effectively.

Studies have also shown that physical activity can decrease insulin resistance, which improves glucose tolerance in people with diabetes. A lack of exercise, therefore, can exacerbate glucose metabolism issues and may lead to complications in the long run.

Did you know that your genes may hold the key to your glucose metabolism, too? Research has shown that certain genes can increase the likelihood of developing insulin resistance, leading to high blood sugar levels over time. Having a family history of diabetes puts you at a higher risk of developing glucose metabolism issues, and it's something that you should keep in mind when managing your condition.

Chronic stress is another important factor that can wreak havoc on your glucose metabolism. When your body is under stress, it releases stress hormones such as cortisol and adrenaline, which can cause an increase in blood sugar levels. Over time, chronic stress can impair your body's response to insulin and may lead to insulin resistance, which affects your glucose metabolism.

Finally, certain medications can also affect your glucose metabolism. Drugs such as corticosteroids (pain and inflammation), diuretics (water pill), and beta-blockers (heart and blood pressure) have all been known to cause glucose metabolism issues, either by increasing insulin resistance or by impairing your body's ability to produce insulin.

So, if you're taking any medications that may be affecting your blood sugar levels, it's crucial to talk to your doctor about possible alternatives or adjustments.

CARBS AND DIABETES

When you have diabetes, controlling your blood sugar levels is essential to maintaining your overall health. One of the critical considerations is how many carbohydrates you consume every day. Carbohydrates (carbs) are broken down into sugar in the body.

Despite the many myths about carbs and diabetes, they're not enemies! In fact, they are essential for providing energy to your body and keeping it running smoothly. But just like with every food, it's essential to calculate your carb intake and choose the right type of carbs.

Let's take a closer look.

What Are Carbs?

Macronutrients include protein, fats, and carbs; these are the main sources of fuel that allow your body to function. Carbohydrates provide glucose, which is the primary energy source for your body. Carbohydrates are found in many foods, including grains, fruits, vegetables, and beans.

When you eat carbs, your body converts them into glucose, which your cells use for energy. It's essential to maintain an adequate supply of carbs and control your blood glucose levels at the same time.

How Do Carbs Fit Into a Healthy Diet?

Carbs are an essential part of a healthy diet, but it's crucial to choose the right type of carbs, such as whole grains, fruits, vegetables, and beans, rather than refined carbs like pastries, candies, and white bread.

Now, that's not to say that you must ban bread entirely. You just need to set limits. Scot Lester, who was diagnosed with diabetes in 2012, found that he was able to continue eating carbohydrates as long as he limited himself to just 35 grams per day (a challenge, still, since he was a self-described sweet tooth).

Roger Hare is another example. When he wants to splurge, he tests his blood sugar levels first. If they're lower, he allows himself a bit more carbs - if not, he limits it. This helps him stay in tune with what his body needs.

You should aim to include carbohydrates in every meal or snack, but don't overdo it. One way to calculate your daily carb intake is by talking to your healthcare professional or even better, a nutritionist. They will help you determine the number of carbs you should consume daily based on your age, weight, and other factors.

Types of Carbohydrates

Let's break down carbs even more! There are three types of carbohydrates: sugars, starches, and fiber.

Sugars are the simplest type of carb, found in many foods such as fruits, syrups, and honey. Starches are a complex type of carb that the body breaks down into glucose, found in grains, potatoes, and legumes.

The third type of carb is fiber, which is not digested by the body, found in vegetables, whole grains, and fruits. To maintain healthy blood sugar levels, choose unrefined and complex carbs whenever you can. Refined carbs are processed whereas unrefined contain more natural fiber.

Whole and unprocessed carbs (unrefined and complex) include whole grains, beans, fruits, and vegetables. These are all great sources of fiber, vitamins, minerals, and phytonutrients.

Simple and processed carbs (refined and simple) include sugar and processed grains that have been stripped of all bran, fiber, and nutrients such as white bread, white flour, pizza dough, pasta, pastries, desserts, white rice and often breakfast cereals.

Net Carbs and Glycemic Index

The concept of net carbs was introduced to help people with diabetes manage their carb intake. Net carbs are the total number of carbohydrates in a food minus the fiber content that the body doesn't digest. A food that has a lot of carbohydrates but also has a lot of fiber will have fewer net carbs than one that has the same amount of carbohydrates, but less fiber.

The glycemic index (GI) is another term used for carbohydrates. It's a scale that measures how quickly a particular food raises blood sugar levels.

Foods with a high glycemic index rank high on the scale, and those with a low glycemic index rank low. Foods with a lower glycemic index are usually better for people with diabetes since they don't cause a sudden spike in blood sugar levels.

High glycemic index foods include white bread, white rice, breakfast cereals and cereal bars, cakes, cookies, potatoes, fries, chips, some fruits such as watermelon and pineapple, and sweetened yogurt.

Low glycemic index foods include green vegetables, most fruits, raw carrots, kidney beans, chickpeas, and lentils.

Don't get too caught up in the terminology, this is just to give you an idea in case your medical provider or nutritionist mentions these terms.

How Many Carbs Do You Need?

The number of carbohydrates you need varies based on your age, weight, gender, and activity level.

Most people require an intake of at least 130 grams a day. A pro marathon runner might eat more than 500 grams of carbohydrates, while someone who is inactive might need as little as 50.

However, when you have diabetes, you would need to regulate your intake of carbs due to its impact on blood sugar levels. That's why you will want to consult with your dietitian or diabetes educator to help you determine the right amount of carbs per day for you.

Carbohydrates and Your Health

Raise your hand if you have ever been at a restaurant and stare blankly at the menu, trying to figure out which dish has the least amount of carbs. Or you've experienced that dreaded feeling when you prick your finger to check your blood sugar, only to see the numbers jump after consuming a high-carb meal.

As a diabetic, you need to be cautious of the amount and type of carbs we consume because our bodies do not produce enough insulin or can't use it properly to regulate our blood sugar levels.

It is important to remember that everyone's body processes carbs differently. What might cause a spike in your blood sugar might not have the same effect on someone else. Keep track of the foods you eat and monitor your blood sugar levels to see how certain foods affect you personally.

Choosing Your Carbohydrates Wisely

Now, when it comes to choosing your carbs wisely, there are a few things to keep in mind. First, aim for complex carbohydrates instead of simple carbohydrates.

Complex carbs, again, take longer to digest, providing a slower release of glucose into the bloodstream, which helps prevent blood sugar spikes. Good sources of complex carbs include sweet potatoes, brown rice, quinoa, and legumes. On the other hand, simple carbs such as candy, soda, and white bread are quickly broken down into glucose, causing a rapid rise in blood sugar levels.

Another crucial factor to consider is portion size. While it is important to be mindful of the type of carbs you're consuming, the amount you eat can also impact your blood sugar levels. Try to stick to recommended serving sizes for foods that contain carbs and be mindful of portion sizes when dining out.

Remember that not all carbs are equal. Foods with a high GI (glycemic index) score (such as white bread and sugary drinks) cause a rapid spike in blood sugar, whole foods with a low GI score (such as most fruits and vegetables) have a slower effect on blood sugar levels. Aim for foods with a lower GI score to help keep your blood sugar levels steady.

HOW INSULIN RESISTANCE OCCURS

Insulin resistance is a condition that impairs your body's ability to use insulin, a hormone that helps regulate blood sugar levels. It's a common problem among people with type 2 diabetes, but it can also affect those with type 1 diabetes and other health conditions as well.

To understand insulin resistance, let's quickly recap how insulin works in the body. Insulin is produced by the pancreas and helps your body use glucose (sugar) from the food you eat for energy.

When you eat, your body releases insulin to help move glucose from your bloodstream into your cells. Think of insulin as a key that unlocks the door to your cells, allowing glucose to enter.

However, if you have insulin resistance, your cells become resistant to the effects of insulin. This means that your body needs to produce more insulin to get the same amount of glucose into your cells. Over time, this can lead to high insulin levels in the bloodstream, which can cause a range of health problems, including type 2 diabetes, heart disease, and obesity.

There are several factors that can contribute to insulin resistance, including genetics, lifestyle, and body weight. For example, if you have a family history of diabetes or are overweight, you may be more likely to develop insulin resistance.

Similarly, a sedentary lifestyle and a diet high in processed and sugary foods can also increase your risk.

Fortunately, there are several steps you can take to manage insulin resistance and improve your overall health.

One of the most effective strategies is to make lifestyle changes, such as exercising regularly and eating a healthy diet that's low in sugar and refined carbohydrates. This can help your body become more sensitive to insulin, reducing the need for high insulin levels.

I'll give you more tips later in this book but know that medication can also be prescribed to help manage insulin resistance. These medications work by increasing insulin sensitivity or reducing insulin resistance in the body. They are usually prescribed in combination with lifestyle changes and can be very effective in controlling blood sugar levels and preventing diabetes complications.

THE IMPACT OF HIGH BLOOD SUGAR ON THE BODY

Sugar is in everything we eat, from cakes and sweets to our everyday food choices, like bread and pasta. However, when enjoying sugar in copious quantities, it can become deadly for diabetics.

High blood sugar, or hyperglycemia, occurs when your body cannot produce or use insulin correctly. Again, insulin is responsible for maintaining your blood sugar levels. If left untreated, high blood sugar can cause damage to your body's vital organs, such as your heart, kidneys, and eyes. And it can cause neurological problems like numbness and tingling in the extremities.

Moderate to severe cases of high blood sugar can lead to a condition called diabetic ketoacidosis. This happens when your body starts breaking down fat for energy instead of glucose and leads to the production of ketones.

Ketones are like acids that accumulate in the blood. They can cause severe damage to your blood vessels and lead to low blood pressure, a rapid heartbeat, and even coma.

While high blood sugar can go unnoticed in its initial stages, some telltale signs include fatigue, dry mouth, increased thirst, frequent urination, and headaches. Other symptoms include blurred vision, nerve damage, loss of consciousness, and even heart attack.

To manage high blood sugar levels, you need to commit to a healthy lifestyle. It includes a healthy diet, regular exercise, and taking any prescribed medication. To keep your blood sugar in check, you will need to control your carbohydrate intake, stay hydrated, and monitor your glucose levels regularly. Taking medication as prescribed and adjusting it according to your doctor's recommendations can help control your blood sugar levels.

It can be challenging to manage high blood sugar levels without support. That is why having a good support system is essential. You can seek support from diabetes support groups, family, friends, and even healthcare professionals.

Together, you can manage your blood sugar levels and avoid complications - and remember, you have a built-in community right here in this book, so stick with me as we go through some lifestyle modifications you can easily make.

THE RELATIONSHIP BETWEEN INSULIN AND BLOOD SUGAR

Again, insulin is a hormone that's produced in the pancreas, a gland located just behind your stomach. Its primary function is to regulate the amount of glucose (sugar) in your bloodstream.

When you eat carbohydrates, your body breaks them down into glucose molecules, which are then transported to your cells by the bloodstream. Insulin allows glucose to enter and be used as energy. Without insulin, glucose would accumulate in your bloodstream, leading to a condition known as hyperglycemia or high blood sugar.

However, in some cases, the body's production of insulin is impaired, leading to the condition we know all too well as diabetes. In type 1 diabetes, the pancreas doesn't produce enough insulin, while in type 2 diabetes, the body becomes resistant to insulin, leading to a buildup of glucose in the bloodstream.

To manage diabetes, diabetics may need to inject synthetic insulin or take medications that enhance the body's response to insulin.

While insulin is essential for regulating blood sugar, too much of it can also be harmful. When you eat a large meal or consume too many carbohydrates, your body releases a surge of insulin to deal with the excess glucose. This can cause your blood sugar levels to drop rapidly, leading to a condition known as hypoglycemia or low blood sugar.

Symptoms of hypoglycemia include dizziness, confusion, sweating, and even loss of consciousness in severe cases. To avoid hypoglycemia, diabetics may need to monitor their blood sugar levels frequently and adjust their medication or food intake accordingly.

The relationship between insulin and blood sugar is dynamic and complex, with many factors influencing their interaction.

For diabetics, understanding how insulin affects their blood sugar levels is crucial to managing their condition. Whether you're newly diagnosed or have been living with diabetes for years, it's never too late to educate yourself about your body's inner workings. Hopefully, this chapter has helped you to do just that!

Now that you know what glucose and insulin are, you hopefully have a better understanding of how your body works - and what can go wrong.

In the next chapter, we'll explore the root causes of diabetes and how these root causes can exacerbate the problem if they aren't properly managed. It might be overwhelming, but knowing about all the different variables that are at play can make a huge difference in managing your symptoms.

Ready to get started? Keep reading to learn more…

3

THE CAUSES AND PREVENTION OF DIABETES

"Diabetes sounds like you're going to die when you hear it. I was immediately frightened. But once I got a better idea of what it was and that it was something I could manage myself, I was comforted."

— NICK JONAS

Diabetes. It's a word that can leave people feeling frightened and helpless. It can seem like a death sentence, but it's important to remember that people with diabetes can still lead long, healthy lives.

The key is understanding the causes of diabetes and taking steps to prevent them from derailing you.

Now that you know what diabetes is, we need to take a closer look at some of the causes. While the exact causes of both Type 1 and Type 2 diabetes are not fully understood, there are several factors that can increase your risk, especially when they exist together.

Let's take a closer look.

WHAT GENETIC FACTORS CONTRIBUTE TO DIABETES?

One of the strongest predictors of type 2 diabetes is having a family history of the disease. If a close relative, such as a parent or sibling, has the condition, your risk of developing it increases. This is because type 2 diabetes has a significant genetic component.

Scientists have identified several genes that are associated with type 2 diabetes risk, including TCF7L2, CDKAL1, HHEX, and FTO. These genes are involved in regulating insulin production and glucose metabolism, and variations in their DNA sequences can lead to impaired insulin secretion and increased insulin resistance.

Another important factor that affects type 2 diabetes risk is ethnicity. Certain ethnic groups, such as African Americans, Hispanics, Native Americans, and Asian Americans, are more likely to develop the condition than others.

This is partly due to genetic differences that affect insulin sensitivity and glucose metabolism. For example, African Americans and Hispanics tend to have a higher prevalence of the TCF7L2 gene variant, which is associated with a higher risk of type 2 diabetes.

By contrast, Native Americans have a higher prevalence of genetic variants that affect lipid metabolism (cholesterol), which can increase their risk of developing diabetes.

Obesity is a major risk factor for type 2 diabetes, and genetics can also play a role in this relationship. Researchers have identified certain genetic variants that are associated with higher body mass index (BMI) and increased adiposity (fat mass).

These variants can affect the regulation of appetite, energy expenditure, and lipid metabolism, all of which can contribute to the development of obesity and type 2 diabetes. Some of the genes that have been implicated in this process include FTO, MC4R, and PPARG.

In addition to DNA sequences, epigenetic modifications also play a role in the development of type 2 diabetes. Epigenetics refers to changes in gene expression that do not involve alterations to the DNA sequence itself. Nutrition and food sources have an impact on epigenetics (gene expression).

Factors such as diet, exercise, and environmental toxins can all influence epigenetic modifications and affect the risk of diabetes. For example, studies have shown that maternal exposure to a high-fat diet during pregnancy can alter the epigenetic marks on the offspring's DNA, leading to increased diabetes risk later in life.

Finally, it is important to recognize that the relationship between genetics and type 2 diabetes is complex and multifaceted. In many cases, genetic factors may only increase the risk of diabetes under certain environmental conditions.

For example, individuals with a high genetic risk of diabetes may only develop the disease if they also lead a sedentary lifestyle or consume a diet high in sugar and fat. By contrast, those with a low genetic risk may still develop diabetes if they are exposed to certain environmental risk factors.

WHICH LIFESTYLE CHOICES IMPACT DIABETES RISK?

Let's focus on the lifestyle choices that can impact diabetes risk and what you can do to decrease your risk.

Food

The food you eat plays a big role in your risk of developing diabetes. Eating a diet that is high in sugar, refined carbohydrates, and unhealthy fats can all contribute to an increased risk of diabetes.

On the other hand, a diet that is rich in fruits, vegetables, whole grains, and lean protein can help lower your risk. Be mindful of your food choices by reading nutrition labels and aiming for a balanced diet.

Exercise

Regular exercise is also important when it comes to reducing your risk of diabetes. Exercise helps to improve insulin sensitivity, which means your cells are better able to use insulin to process glucose. This can help to keep blood sugar levels within a healthy range.

Even just 30 minutes of physical activity per day can make a big difference in reducing your risk of diabetes. The recommended minimum goal is 150 minutes per week.

Medication

If you already have diabetes, it's important to take your medication as prescribed by your healthcare provider. This can help to keep your blood sugar levels under control and reduce your risk of complications.

Make sure to talk to your healthcare provider if you have any concerns about taking your medication.

Illness

Certain illnesses, such as high blood pressure, heart disease, and obesity, can increase your risk of diabetes. By managing any existing health conditions, you have, you can reduce your risk of developing diabetes. This includes maintaining a healthy weight, eating a balanced diet, and exercising regularly.

Alcohol

Drinking alcohol in moderation is okay, but not recommended, for people with diabetes. However, excessive drinking can increase your risk of developing diabetes - so it should be avoided. If you choose to drink alcohol, do so in moderation and make sure to eat food with your drink.

Menstruation and Menopause

For women, hormonal changes during menstruation and menopause can affect blood sugar levels. It's important for women with diabetes to stay on top of these changes and work with their healthcare provider to manage their diabetes. This may involve adjusting medication doses or monitoring blood sugar levels more closely during these times.

OTHER RISK FACTORS FOR DIABETES

Although the factors listed above are some of the most often-cited reasons for why people develop type 2 diabetes, they certainly aren't the only ones. Here are a few more.

Obesity

As mentioned, being overweight is a well-known risk factor for type 2 diabetes.

However, it's not just about the total number of pounds a person carries, but also about where that weight is distributed.

Carrying extra weight in the midsection or having a high waist-to-hip ratio, increases the risk of developing diabetes. This is because abdominal fat produces chemicals that can interfere with the body's ability to produce insulin, the hormone responsible for regulating blood sugar levels.

If you have a large waist circumference, losing even a small amount of weight can help improve your blood sugar control.

Age

As we get older, the risk of developing diabetes increases. This is partly due to lifestyle factors, such as decreased physical activity, poorer dietary choices, and weight gain. However, there may also be genetic factors at play.

The incidence of diabetes increases significantly after age 45, with most cases occurring in those over 65. If you fall into this age range, it's important to be vigilant about monitoring your blood sugar levels and adhering to a healthy lifestyle to help prevent or manage diabetes.

Sedentary Lifestyle

Leading a sedentary lifestyle, characterized by little to no physical activity, is another risk factor for diabetes. Exercise helps the body use insulin more efficiently, which in turn helps to regulate blood sugar levels.

On the other hand, a lack of exercise can cause insulin resistance, which makes it harder for the body to use insulin effectively. This risk factor is especially relevant for those who have a family history of diabetes or other related conditions. If you're not currently active, talk to your doctor about how to start a safe and effective exercise regimen.

Family History

If you have a family member with diabetes, your own risk of developing the condition is higher.

However, it's important to note that family history is just one of many risk factors and does not automatically guarantee a diabetes diagnosis.

Still, having a close relative with diabetes (especially a parent or sibling) can make it more important to manage other risk factors, such as weight, blood pressure, and cholesterol levels. It's also important to stay on top of regular diabetes screenings and to be aware of any early symptoms that may arise.

THE ROLE OF SLEEP AND STRESS IN DIABETES PREVENTION

Diet and exercise are typical measures used to manage the condition. However, what most people don't realize is that sleep and stress play a crucial role in diabetes prevention as well.

Lack of sleep or poor-quality sleep can contribute to the development of type 2 diabetes in several ways. For starters, it can lead to insulin resistance and an increased risk of type 2 diabetes.

Studies have shown that people who sleep less than six hours per night have a higher risk of developing type 2 diabetes than those who sleep more. Also, poor sleep can affect our stress hormone levels, leading to insulin resistance, inflammation, and obesity.

Chronic stress can increase your risk of developing diabetes. This is because stress hormones can cause an increase in blood sugar levels. To manage stress, try activities such as yoga, meditation, or deep breathing exercises. Stress levels can have a direct impact on your blood sugar levels. Chronic stress can lead to insulin resistance, which could ultimately result in type 2 diabetes. Cortisol, the stress hormone, raises blood sugar levels, making it difficult to manage the condition.

STEROID USE AND DIABETES

If you've used steroids or are currently using steroids, you might be curious about how they will come into play in terms of managing your diabetes.

What Are Steroids?

Steroids are synthetic substances that are designed to mimic the effects of the hormone testosterone.

They are commonly used in medicine to treat hormonal issues, muscle loss, and to trigger muscle growth. Steroids can be taken orally, injected, or applied topically to the skin. They also come in different forms, such as creams, gels, and sprays.

The two main types of steroids are corticosteroids and anabolic steroids. Corticosteroids are typically used for treating inflammation or autoimmune diseases, such as asthma and lupus.

They work by reducing inflammation in the body and, in turn, easing symptoms. Anabolic steroids, on the other hand, are used to build muscle mass and strength, which is often the reason why people who work out use them.

How Steroids Impact Blood Glucose Levels

Steroids are known to increase blood glucose levels as they affect the way your body metabolizes sugar.

Normally, the body produces insulin to help regulate blood sugar levels. However, when you take steroids, this can lead to insulin resistance, which can cause elevated blood sugars. Steroids can also cause the liver to release stored glucose into the bloodstream, further increasing blood glucose levels.

If you're taking steroids and notice an increase in your blood glucose levels, it's essential to speak with your doctor. They may recommend taking extra insulin or other medications to help regulate your blood sugars.

It's also important to note that not all steroids are equal when it comes to their impact on blood glucose levels. Some steroids, such as dexamethasone, have more significant impacts on blood glucose levels than others. Again, it's essential to speak with your doctor about the steroid you're taking and what you can do to help manage blood glucose level changes.

Diabetes Management When You Must Use Steroids

Steroids can affect glucose levels and insulin sensitivity, which is why it's essential to keep an eye on your diabetes management when taking them.

Check Glucose Levels More Often

Steroids can affect glucose levels, so it's essential to monitor them more frequently than usual. Frequent testing will help you catch any potential issues before they become a problem. If you find that your glucose levels are consistently higher than normal, speak to your healthcare team about adjusting your insulin dosage or medication.

Increase Insulin or Medication Dosage Based on Doctor Recommendations

If you're taking insulin or other diabetes medications, it may be necessary to adjust your dosage when taking steroids. Talk to your healthcare provider about increasing your insulin or medication dosage, as they may advise you to take more.

Don't take it upon yourself to adjust your insulin dosage without consulting your healthcare team, as it can lead to serious complications.

Monitor Urine and Blood Ketones

When taking steroids, your body may start producing ketones, which can be dangerous if left unchecked. Ketones are commonly found in individuals with type 1 diabetes, but individuals with type 2 diabetes can also develop them if their glucose levels are consistently high.

Monitoring your urine and blood ketones is crucial when taking steroids. Speak to your healthcare team about how to do this effectively, and what you should do if your levels become too high.

Now that you know some of the underlying causes of diabetes, it is time to move on - you know what the problem is, so how do you deal with it?

In the next few chapters, we will give you an overview of some of the options that are available to help you treat and manage your diabetes. We will start first with the broad options before we establish more specific steps you can take.

4

TREATMENT OPTIONS FOR DIABETES

"Think about it: heart disease and diabetes account for more deaths in the U.S. and worldwide than everything else combined. They are completely preventable through lifestyle habits without drugs or surgery."

— DEAN ORNISH

Being diagnosed with diabetes can be overwhelming, especially when it comes to figuring out the best treatment options available. Luckily, the medical community has made incredible strides in recent years, offering a plethora of ways to control and manage this chronic illness.

Insulin is great. With over a hundred years of use, insulin is one of the most reliable and effective treatment options for diabetes.

However, it's certainly not the only option. With the right treatment plan and medical guidance, diabetes doesn't have to hold you back from living your best life.

Here are some of the other treatment options for diabetes so that you have plenty of information at your disposal when you meet with your doctor.

LIFESTYLE CHANGES AS A FIRST-LINE TREATMENT

The good news is that there are many things you can do to manage your type 2 diabetes - without medication. While there is no substitution for the right medication when you truly need it, that medication will be significantly more effective if you combine it with certain lifestyle adjustments.

A patient from Johns Hopkins who was diagnosed with diabetes at age 50 says "It's a lifestyle change – it impacts every part of your life (medications, meals, etc.). If you can realize this earlier on, you'll get under control much more quickly."

One of the most important lifestyle changes you can make when you have diabetes is to eat a healthy, balanced diet. This means avoiding sugary and processed foods and opting for lean proteins, whole grains, and plenty of fruits and vegetables.

Exercise is another important lifestyle change that can help manage diabetes. Regular physical activity can improve insulin sensitivity, which can help lower your blood sugar levels.

Maintaining a healthy weight is important for people with diabetes because excess body fat can make it more difficult for the body to use insulin effectively. Losing just a few pounds can improve insulin sensitivity and help lower your blood sugar levels.

Stress can cause a rise in blood sugar levels, making it important to find ways to manage stress effectively. Whether it's through meditation, deep breathing, or spending time with friends and family, finding ways to reduce stress can help improve your overall wellbeing and help manage diabetes.

And finally, it's important to monitor your blood sugar levels regularly to make sure they're within a healthy range. Your doctor can advise you on how often you should check your blood sugar levels and what your target range should be.

MEDICATION FOR BLOOD SUGAR CONTROL

Apart from making necessary changes in diet and exercise, medication plays a significant role in keeping blood sugar levels in check. With a wide range of medications available in the market, it can be quite daunting to choose which best suits your needs.

Here are some of the most common options that might be prescribed.

Metformin

Metformin is one of the most prescribed medications for blood sugar control. It works by reducing glucose production in the liver and enhancing insulin sensitivity. The advantages of metformin include reduced risk of hypoglycemia, improved cholesterol levels, and modest weight loss. The disadvantage of metformin is that it can cause digestive side effects such as nausea, vomiting, diarrhea, and stomach cramps. Metformin also depletes vitamin B12 which often requires supplementation.

Sulfonylureas

Sulfonylureas are oral medications that stimulate the pancreas to produce and release more insulin. They are generally inexpensive and effective in lowering blood sugar levels. Sulfonylureas are associated with an increased risk of hypoglycemia, weight gain, and cardiovascular side effects in some people. Examples include glipizide, glyburide, and glimepiride.

Thiazolidinediones (TZDs)

TZDs are oral medications that improve insulin sensitivity and reduce glucose production in the liver. They are typically used in conjunction with other medications and can cause fluid retention, weight gain, and an increased risk of heart failure. Examples include rosiglitazone and pioglitazone.

Dipeptidyl peptidase-4 inhibitors (DPP-4 inhibitors)

DPP-4 inhibitors are oral medications that help lower blood sugar levels by preventing the breakdown of a hormone called glucagon-like peptide-1 (GLP-1).

The advantages of DPP-4 inhibitors include a lower risk of hypoglycemia, weight neutrality, and a lower risk of cardiovascular side effects. They can cause upper respiratory tract infections, headaches, and gastrointestinal side effects.

These medications are often expensive because generics are not available. These include Januvia (sitagliptin), Onglyza (saxagliptin), Tradjenta (linagliptin), and Nesina (alogliptin).

GLP-1 receptor agonists

GLP-1 receptor agonists are injectable medications that mimic the effects of GLP-1 and help lower blood sugar levels. They also reduce appetite, promote weight loss, and have a lower risk of hypoglycemia.

The disadvantage of GLP-1 receptor agonists is that they are expensive, require injections, and can cause gastrointestinal side effects such as nausea, vomiting, and diarrhea.

These medications are often expensive because generics are not available. These include Trulicity (dulaglutide), Bydureon (Exenatide) weekly, and Byetta (Exenatide) twice daily, Ozempic (semaglutide), Victoza (liraglutide), Wegovy (semaglutide) and Rybelsus (semaglutide). Rybelsus is the only drug in this class that is a tablet taken by mouth.

SGLT2 Inhibitors

SGLT2 inhibitors are another newer type of medication that work by blocking the reabsorption of glucose in the kidneys and increasing its excretion in the urine. This results in lower blood sugar levels and weight loss.

SGLT2 inhibitors have a low risk of hypoglycemia but can cause genital infections and increase the risk of dehydration and kidney problems.

Meglitinides

Meglitinides are a type of oral medication used to control blood sugar levels in people with type 2 diabetes. They work by stimulating the pancreas to secrete more insulin, which helps reduce blood sugar levels.

Meglitinides are often prescribed in combination with other diabetes medications such as Metformin and Insulin. Drugs in the Meglitinides class are usually taken before meals to help prevent high blood sugar spikes that typically occur after eating.

Meglitinides are beneficial to people who have undergone surgery, and those who can't control their blood sugar levels through lifestyle modifications alone. One major advantage of

Meglitinides over other diabetes medications is that they have a shorter duration of action. This means that they are processed more quickly by the body, and therefore have a lower risk of causing low blood sugar levels (hypoglycemia).

Mounjaro

Mounjaro is a new medication that combines two hormones called GIP and GLP-1. GIP stimulates insulin production in response to food, while GLP-1 helps to regulate blood sugar levels and decrease appetite.

This medication has shown promising results in clinical trials for people with type 2 diabetes, including improved blood sugar control and weight loss.

THE IMPORTANCE OF INSULIN THERAPY

One treatment option that has been known to bring incredible relief to people with type 2 diabetes is insulin therapy. Despite its obvious benefits, many people shy away from insulin therapy due to common myths and misconceptions surrounding its use.

Insulin therapy may be recommended as a standalone or in combination with other diabetes medications to achieve better glycemic control. The most common reason why people with type 2 diabetes decline insulin therapy is the misconception that it is only reserved for severe cases.

While insulin treatment may indeed be necessary for people with severe cases, insulin resistance can occur in anyone, regardless of symptom severity. In fact, starting insulin therapy earlier on in the illness can help achieve better glycemic control and improve long-term outcomes.

Another common myth about insulin therapy is the fear of needles. While it is understandable to feel anxious about self-injecting insulin, the reality is that needle technology has come a long way, and it is now easier and less painful to use insulin pens than it was before.

Furthermore, insulin injections are necessary for keeping blood sugar levels in check and can be an important aspect of diabetes management. Your medical practitioner will work with you to help you feel comfortable using the insulin pen and can suggest means of reducing discomfort during the injection process, such as numbing creams and adjusting injection sites.

Insulin therapy presents some unique benefits for people with type 2 diabetes, such as its ability to help regulate blood sugar levels dramatically. Insulin is created naturally by the pancreas and is used by your body to turn glucose into energy. In people with diabetes, however, the pancreas does not produce enough insulin or stops producing insulin altogether, causing blood glucose levels to soar. Insulin therapy can help compensate for the low or no insulin production demands of your body.

It is important to note that while insulin therapy is powerful, it should never replace a healthy diet and an active lifestyle. Combining insulin therapy with healthy lifestyle habits can lead to optimal results. Often lifestyle changes can result in decreasing medication requirements and enable your pancreas to regain function.

HOW, WHEN, AND WHY - MONITORING BLOOD SUGAR LEVELS

Monitoring blood sugar levels is extremely important for people who have type 2 diabetes.

It is a crucial aspect of diabetes control and can help prevent complications such as nerve damage, kidney disease, and blindness.

Let's take a closer look at how and why you should do this.

How and When to Test Your Blood Sugar

The first step to monitoring blood glucose levels is talking to your healthcare provider. They will recommend the frequency of testing based on your medical history and current diabetes management plan.

Some people with type 2 diabetes may need to test their blood sugar level multiple times a day, while others only need to do it once a week or as recommended by their doctor.

Daily Finger Sticks

The most common way to test blood glucose levels is through daily finger sticks. This involves pricking your finger with a small needle called a lancet and collecting a drop of blood onto a test strip.

The test strip is then inserted into a glucose meter, which will provide a reading of your blood glucose level. This is an affordable and straightforward method but can be quite painful due to frequent punctures.

Continuous Monitors

Advancements in technology have led to continuous glucose monitoring (CGM), which provides real-time glucose readings. A CGM device is inserted under the skin, and a sensor measures glucose levels in the fluid between cells. The readings are displayed on a monitor, providing a constant stream of information and a more comprehensive picture of blood glucose levels.

Further, some CGMs alert their users to changes in glucose levels when they are high, low, or fluctuating, assuring timely intervention from the health-care providers. Examples include Dexcom and Freestyle Libre.

However, CGM is relatively expensive and may not be covered by all insurance providers, while some people find the process of inserting and removing the device from their body uncomfortable.

What is Considered Normal Glucose?

First, a quick review about what glucose is. Glucose is a type of sugar that comes from the foods we eat. When glucose enters our blood, it's called blood glucose or blood sugar. It's the primary source of energy for our bodies, but too much of it can be harmful. That's why it's essential to keep our blood sugar levels within a healthy range.

What Numbers Should You See?

The normal glucose range is between 70-99 mg/dL when fasting. This means your blood was drawn after you haven't eaten for 8-12 hours.

What is Fasting and What Are Post Prandial Blood Sugar Levels?

Your blood sugar naturally rises after eating. How high it goes and how long it stays there depend on various factors, such as what you ate, how much you ate, and how fast your body digests food.

The normal postprandial blood sugar range is less than 140 mg/dL two hours after eating. However, the American Diabetes Association recommends keeping your postprandial levels under 180 mg/dL.

When Should You Be Concerned?

If your blood sugar levels are higher than the normal range, you could be at risk for complications such as kidney damage, nerve damage, blindness, heart disease, and stroke. But when should you be concerned?

The best piece of advice is to pay attention to your symptoms. If you feel thirsty, fatigued, have blurry vision, or experience frequent urination, that could indicate high blood sugar levels. You should also talk to your healthcare provider, who can help you understand your numbers and develop a plan to manage your blood sugar levels.

What is Hemoglobin A1C?

Hemoglobin A1C is a blood test that measures the amount of glucose (sugar) that has attached to hemoglobin, a protein in your red blood cells. The test gives you a picture of your average blood sugar levels over the past two to three months, rather than just at one moment in time.

That's important because blood sugar levels can fluctuate throughout the day, depending on what you eat, your physical activity, and other factors. By measuring your HbA1C, you and your healthcare team can get a better idea of how well your diabetes is being managed over time.

Normal Values and Goals

HbA1C levels are expressed as a percentage of the total hemoglobin in your blood. The higher the percentage, the higher your average blood glucose levels have been.

For people without diabetes, HbA1C levels are typically between 4 and 5.6%. However, people with type 2 diabetes may have higher levels of HbA1C due to the body's inability to use insulin effectively. The goal for most people with type 2 diabetes is to keep their HbA1C levels below 7%. However, your doctor may set a different target depending on your health status and other factors.

The American Diabetes Association advises people with diabetes to achieve an HbA1C level of 7% or lower, which translates to an average blood glucose level of 154 mg/dL. However, the target range may vary depending on your age, overall health status, and personal preferences.

If you're older or have underlying health concerns, your doctor may suggest a less stringent target range, like 8%. For pregnant women with diabetes, the goal range may also differ. Your healthcare provider will consider your unique circumstances to advise what target HbA1C level is best for you.

While the ADA has general guidelines on HbA1C goals, each patient's needs are unique. Your healthcare team, including your doctor, diabetes educator, and nutritionist, can help you set a customized target HbA1C level that aligns with your specific health status and preferences.

Generally, if you have a history of diabetes complications, your doctor may set a lower target HbA1C level. On the other hand, if you have underlying conditions that can cause hypoglycemia, your doctor may recommend a higher HbA1C range.

High levels of HbA1C over time can cause significant damage to your blood vessels, nerves, and organs. Along with other lifestyle changes and medications, monitoring your HbA1C levels regularly can help you stay on top of your diabetes management and live a healthier life.

Every 1% decrease in HbA1C results in a 40% reduction in the risk of developing diabetes-related complications. Therefore, achieving your target HbA1C goal is critical in preventing or delaying complications of diabetes.

Signs and Symptoms You Might Have Elevated Blood Sugar

When blood sugar levels get too high, it can lead to severe complications, and in some cases, it may lead to an emergency requiring immediate medical attention. Therefore, it's crucial to know the signs and symptoms of elevated blood sugar to act quickly and avoid any severe complications.

Here are some of the most common:

- **Extreme thirst**: You might feel excessively thirsty, and it can be challenging to quench your thirst even if you drink enough water. This symptom indicates that your body is trying to flush out excess sugar via urination, which leads to dehydration.
- **Frequent urination:** If you are urinating more often than usual, it could be due to elevated blood sugar levels. When your body's cells cannot absorb glucose efficiently, the kidneys try to flush it out of your system via increased urination.
- **Fatigue**: Elevated blood sugar levels can lead to fatigue because your cells are not getting enough glucose. As a result, you may experience feelings of tiredness and lack of energy.
- **Blurred vision:** High blood sugar levels can affect the tiny blood vessels in your eyes, leading to blurred or distorted vision. If you experience any changes in vision, along with other symptoms of high blood sugar, it's essential to seek medical attention.
- **Abdominal pain and vomiting**: If your blood sugar levels are severely elevated, you might experience abdominal pain, nausea, and vomiting. This situation could lead to diabetic ketoacidosis, a potentially life-threatening condition that requires immediate medical attention.

When To Go to the ER

If you experience any of the above symptoms, and they are severe and persistent, you should seek medical attention immediately.

The same advice applies if your blood sugar levels are above 240 mg/dL. At that point, it's crucial to seek medical attention. High blood sugar levels can lead to severe complications such as diabetic coma, which requires urgent medical attention. Make sure you have a plan in place in case of an emergency and know when to seek medical attention.

Signs and Symptoms of Low Blood Sugar

Managing diabetes requires a delicate balance of blood sugar levels, and when those levels drop too low, it can lead to hypoglycemia, or low blood sugar. The symptoms of low blood sugar can range from mild to severe, and it is important to recognize them and act before they become dangerous.

When your blood sugar levels are low, some of the initial signs to watch out for are sweating, trembling, and feeling dizzy. You might also feel hungry, anxious, or irritable. It is not uncommon to have a headache or to feel weak or lightheaded.

Some other signs of low blood sugar include:

- **Change in behavior**: As your blood glucose level continues to drop, you might experience sudden changes in speech or behavior, such as confusion or slurred speech. There is also a possibility of mood swings ranging from embarrassment to aggressive behavior. You might feel like a different person.
- **Physical manifestations:** If left unchecked, severe hypoglycemia can cause seizures, loss of consciousness, or even coma. At this stage, you might experience blurred or double vision. You might appear confused to others and even start making poor judgments, like being unable to tell left from right.
- **Nighttime hypoglycemia:** Low blood sugar can occur at any time of the day or night, but many people with diabetes experience nighttime hypoglycemia. Symptoms of hypoglycemia can wake you up in the middle of the night (nightmares, feeling disoriented) and interfere with your sleep and overall ability to focus. Keep a close eye on nighttime symptoms.

THE IMPORTANCE OF REGULAR MEDICAL CHECK-UPS

Medical check-ups are an essential part of diabetes management. Regular check-ups allow your doctor to monitor your blood sugar levels, blood pressure, and cholesterol.

This can help to prevent or identify complications that may arise from diabetes, such as heart disease, kidney disease, and nerve damage. Your doctor can also identify changes in your health and suggest adjustments to your diabetes management plan to keep you healthy and prevent complications.

Regular medical check-ups give you a chance to discuss any concerns or questions you may have with your doctor. This is an opportunity to review your progress, discuss your treatment plan, and make any necessary changes.

You can discuss any new symptoms you may be experiencing, and your doctor can recommend any necessary tests or referrals. This helps to ensure that you are getting the best possible care and that you are managing your diabetes effectively.

One of the benefits of regular medical check-ups is the opportunity for your doctor to screen for other health conditions that may be related to diabetes.

For example, people with type 2 diabetes are at a higher risk of developing eye conditions, such as diabetic retinopathy.

Regular eye exams can help identify any changes in your vision and prevent damage to your eyes. Your doctor can also screen for other conditions, such as infections and foot problems, which can occur more frequently in people with diabetes.

Regular medical check-ups can also help you to stay motivated and on track with your diabetes management plan.

It can be frustrating and challenging to manage diabetes, but appointments with your doctor can serve as a reminder of the progress you've made and the goals you're working towards. Your doctor can offer guidance and support and can provide you with the tools you need to stay on top of your diabetes management.

Remember that managing diabetes is a lifelong journey—regular medical check-ups are a crucial part of your diabetes management plan.

Now that we've gone over a basic exploration of your options, let's cover in more detail one of the biggest aspects of diabetes management: your diet!

5

MANAGING DIABETES THROUGH DIET

"Good food is wise medicine."

— ALISON LEVITT M.D.

You are what you eat.

There is so much truth to that statement, though of course, it can also be laughable.

You do not become a donut just because you eat a donut, and you don't become a stalk of celery because that's what you choose to snack on, either. That is obvious.

However, what many people do not realize is the major impact that diet has on our overall health. Perhaps nowhere is that truer than for the person with type 2 diabetes.

It is true that managing diabetes can be a challenge, and it's also true that some risk factors for diabetes (like your genetics) are completely out of your control.

But there are some areas in which you have total control — and can take charge of your diabetes symptoms. One of those is your diet.

As the quote above illustrates, the best medicine you can put into your body is the food you choose to nourish it with.

Managing diabetes through diet is all about making healthy choices that work for your situation. Everyone with diabetes is unique, and their dietary needs will differ.

A registered dietitian can help you develop a customized meal plan that includes the right foods in the right proportions, so I do recommend checking in with a nutritionist or dietician for a more personalized plan.

With that said, let's look at some of the most important information about diabetes and your diet so you can make the best and most informed decisions for your needs.

THE ROLE OF CARBOHYDRATES, FATS, AND PROTEINS IN BLOOD SUGAR CONTROL

Carbohydrates are often considered to be the most significant factor in blood sugar control. The carbohydrate in food breaks down into glucose, which is then absorbed into the bloodstream.

The glucose acts as fuel for the body, but in the case of people with diabetes, it can result in high levels of blood sugar.

To manage this, people with diabetes need to ensure that they are consuming the right amount of carbohydrates in their diet and avoiding foods that can spike their blood sugar levels. Ideally, people with diabetes should follow a diet that is low in simple carbohydrates, but high in complex carbohydrates such as whole grains, vegetables, and fruits.

Fats are also a key component in blood sugar control. The right balance of healthy fats can help to decrease insulin resistance and inflammation, leading to improved blood sugar levels.

However, a diet that is high in saturated and trans fats can cause inflammation and lead to insulin resistance, which can be harmful to those with diabetes. Foods that are high in healthy fats include nuts, fatty fish (such as salmon or tuna), avocados, and olive oil.

Protein is vital in maintaining muscle mass and is an excellent source of energy. However, when eating protein, people with diabetes need to exercise caution as it can raise blood sugar levels.

When consuming protein, it is essential to eat smaller portions and to balance it with fiber-rich foods such as vegetables. The best sources of protein for people with diabetes are lean meats, fish, nuts, and legumes.

RECOMMENDED DIETARY GUIDELINES

Again, one of the best ways to manage type 2 diabetes is through proper nutrition. By following recommended dietary guidelines, people with diabetes can maintain healthy blood glucose levels and reduce the risk of diabetes-related complications.

The Importance of Portion Control and Meal Planning

Portion control is key to managing blood glucose levels.

By controlling the amount of carbohydrates, protein, and fat in each meal, people with type 2 diabetes can maintain stable blood sugar levels throughout the day. Shortly, I'll introduce you to "the plate method" to help you balance your meals.

Meal planning is also an essential component of managing diabetes. Planning meals ahead of time can help people stick to their nutrition goals and avoid unhealthy food choices.

Carrying healthy snacks when on-the-go can also help prevent impulse eating and keep blood sugar levels in check.

Strategies for Eating Out and Managing Special Occasions

Eating out and attending special occasions can be challenging for people with diabetes. However, with the right strategies, it is still possible to enjoy meals and events while maintaining healthy blood glucose levels.

When eating out, it's a good idea to check the menu ahead of time and choose restaurants that offer healthy options whenever possible. Pay attention to portion sizes and limit unhealthy extras such as butter, cream, and sugar.

During special occasions such as holidays and family gatherings, it's easy to indulge in unhealthy food options. One way to avoid this is to bring a healthy dish to share. This ensures that there will be at least one healthy option available. It's also important to pace your eating and to avoid going back for seconds.

Widely Accepted Diabetes "Superfoods"

Some foods are considered "superfoods" for people with type 2 diabetes.

What is a "superfood"? It's just a food that has been shown to be particularly beneficial in managing blood glucose levels and reducing the risk of diabetes-related complications. Some of these foods include:

- Non-starchy vegetables such as broccoli, spinach, and kale

- Whole grains such as brown rice, quinoa, and barley
- Lean proteins such as chicken, fish, and tofu
- Nuts and seeds such as almonds, walnuts, and chia seeds
- Healthy fats such as olive oil, avocado, and flaxseed oil

WHAT ABOUT DIETARY SUPPLEMENTS?

As a person with type 2 diabetes, you are likely always searching for ways to manage your condition and keep your blood sugar levels in check. One potential avenue many people explore is the consumption of dietary supplements. But with so many options out there, and conflicting information about their effectiveness, it can be hard to know where to start.

First, let's define what we mean by "dietary supplements." These are products that contain one or more ingredients like vitamins, minerals, herbs, or other botanicals, amino acids, or enzymes.

They're intended to supplement the diet, and come in many forms like capsules, tablets, powders, and drinks. Some dietary supplements are marketed specifically for people with diabetes, claiming to lower blood sugar levels or improve insulin sensitivity.

For instance, magnesium has been shown in some studies to improve insulin sensitivity and glucose control, although the dosage and duration required to have an effect are still unknown.

Similarly, St. John's wort, an herb commonly used to treat depression and anxiety, has been studied for its potential to lower blood sugar levels.

Note that not all supplements are created equal, and some can even be harmful if taken in excess.

For example, high doses of vitamins like A, D, E, and K can accumulate in the body and cause toxic effects. Other supplements may interact with medications like insulin, causing adverse effects.

That is why it's essential to talk to your healthcare provider before taking any supplements, especially if you're using prescription medications or have other health conditions that could be affected.

Another thing to keep in mind is that dietary supplements are not a substitute for a healthy diet and lifestyle. As the name implies, they are meant to supplement your existing routine, not replace it. Eating a balanced diet that is rich in whole grains, fruits and vegetables, lean protein, and healthy fats, combined with regular physical activity, is still the cornerstone of diabetes management.

Finally, it's worth mentioning that dietary supplements can be costly, and insurance may not cover them. It's wise to do some research and compare prices and quality before making a purchase, and to be wary of claims that sound too good to be true.

If you do decide to try a supplement, always choose reputable brands that have been third-party tested for purity and potency and beware of products sold online or in unauthorized retail outlets.

Common supplements used in type 2 diabetes include the following:

- Vitamin B12
- Vitamin D
- Magnesium
- Zinc
- Chromium
- Alpha lipoic acid
- Coenzyme Q10

GUIDANCE ON CREATING YOUR OWN HEALTHY EATING PLAN

A carefully planned diet can help you manage your blood sugar levels, reduce the risk of complications, and improve your overall health. But with so much conflicting information out there, creating your own healthy eating plan can be overwhelming.

Here are some tips.

Why Do You Need to Develop a Healthy Eating Plan?

I'd like to begin by emphasizing why it's so important to develop a healthy eating plan in the first place.

Remember, type 2 diabetes is a chronic condition that occurs when the body becomes resistant to insulin or does not produce enough insulin. Insulin is a hormone that regulates the amount of glucose in your blood.

When your body cannot regulate blood glucose levels effectively, it can lead to a range of complications, including heart disease, stroke, nerve damage, and kidney disease. A healthy eating plan can help you manage your blood sugar levels, control your weight, and reduce your risk of complications.

What Does a Diabetes Diet Involve?

A diabetes diet involves eating a balanced and healthy diet that is low in sugar, saturated and trans fats, cholesterol, and sodium.

This means that you need to limit your intake of processed foods, sugar-sweetened beverages, and high-fat meats. Instead, your diet should consist of nutrient-dense foods, such as vegetables, fruits, whole grains, lean proteins, and healthy fats.

Recommended Foods

The following foods are recommended for people with type 2 diabetes:

- **Vegetables:** Eat a variety of non-starchy vegetables, such as broccoli, spinach, kale, carrots, and peppers.
- **Fruits**: Choose fruits that are low in sugar and high in fiber, such as berries, apples, pears, and oranges.
- **Whole grains:** Choose whole-grain bread, pasta, rice, and cereals.
- **Lean proteins**: Choose lean proteins such as skinless chicken, fish, tofu, and legumes.
- **Healthy fats:** Use olive oil, avocado, nuts, and seeds in moderation.

Foods to Avoid

The following foods should be avoided or limited:

- **Sugary drinks:** Avoid sugar-sweetened beverages such as soda, fruit juice, and sweetened tea.
- **Processed foods:** Limit your intake of processed foods such as white bread, chips, crackers, and cookies.
- **High-fat meats**: Avoid red meat, bacon, sausage, and other high-fat meats.
- **Saturated and trans fats**: Limit your intake of saturated and trans fats found in butter, cheese,

cream, and fried foods.
- **Sodium**: Limit your salt intake to less than 2,300 mg per day.

Putting it All Together: Creating a Plan

Now that you know the basics, how do you create a plan that will help you to coast through any mealtime like a champ? Here are some general ideas that can help you out as you become accustomed to eating a more wholesome, healthful diet.

The Plate Method

The plate method I mentioned earlier is a simple and effective way to plan your meals.

Start by dividing your plate into three sections: half of the plate should be filled with non-starchy vegetables, one quarter with lean protein, and one quarter with grains or starchy vegetables.

This method ensures that you have a balanced meal with carbohydrates, protein, and fiber. You can also add a small serving of fruit or dairy as a snack.

Counting Carbohydrates

Counting carbohydrates is another way to manage your blood sugar levels. Carbohydrates are essential for energy, but some types of carbohydrates can cause a spike in blood sugar levels.

It's important to choose carbohydrates that are high in fiber and avoid refined carbohydrates.

You can start by aiming for 45-60 grams of carbohydrates per meal. A registered dietitian can help you create a personalized meal plan based on your individual needs.

Choose Your Foods

When creating your healthy eating plan, focus on whole foods and avoid processed foods. Whole foods are nutrient-dense and provide your body with essential vitamins and minerals.

Processed foods, on the other hand, are often high in added sugars, sodium, and unhealthy fats. Aim for a variety of colorful vegetables, lean protein, healthy fats, and whole grains.

Glycemic Index

The glycemic index is a ranking system that measures how quickly foods raise blood sugar levels.

Foods with a high glycemic index can cause a spike in blood sugar, whole foods with a low glycemic index can help maintain a steady blood sugar level.

Choose foods with a low glycemic index, such as non-starchy vegetables, whole grains, and legumes. Avoid foods with a high glycemic index, such as processed foods, sugary drinks, and refined carbohydrates.

PUTTING TOGETHER A BASIC MENU PLAN

Need some help putting together a basic menu plan? Here's a sample of one you can use to help you guide your decisions day to day.

Remember, this isn't a "must-do" menu — it's simply some suggestions and ideas to help get you started. You can swap out these foods for ones you like, or ones you prefer to include in your diet for other reasons (for example, getting rid of the milk because you're dairy-free).

Day 1:
Breakfast: Omelet with spinach, mushrooms, and tomatoes (306 calories)
Lunch: Turkey wrap with avocado, lettuce, and tomato on a whole wheat tortilla (342 calories)
Dinner: Grilled chicken breast with steamed vegetables and brown rice (412 calories)
Snack: Greek yogurt with berries (180 calories)

Day 2:
Breakfast: Whole wheat toast with peanut butter and banana (389 calories)
Lunch: Salad with grilled shrimp, mixed greens, cherry tomatoes, and avocado (388 calories)
Dinner: Baked salmon filet with roasted asparagus and quinoa (465 calories)
Snack: Apple slices with almond butter (172 calories)

Day 3:

Breakfast: Greek yogurt with chia seeds and mixed berries (215 calories)

Lunch: Grilled chicken breast with mixed greens and cherry tomatoes (284 calories)

Dinner: Spaghetti squash with turkey bolognese sauce (345 calories)

Snack: Hard-boiled egg with carrot sticks (134 calories)

Day 4:

Breakfast: Oatmeal with sliced banana and cinnamon (268 calories)

Lunch: Tuna salad with mixed greens and avocado (321 calories)

Dinner: Pan-seared pork chops with roasted Brussels sprouts and sweet potato (471 calories)

Snack: Hummus with carrot and celery sticks (152 calories)

Day 5:

Breakfast: Scrambled eggs with cheese and spinach (346 calories)

Lunch: Grilled chicken salad with mixed greens, cherry tomatoes, and balsamic vinaigrette (244 calories)

Dinner: Grilled steak with roasted sweet potatoes and green beans (500 calories)

Snack: Blueberries with a handful of almonds (187 calories)

Day 6:
Breakfast: Veggie breakfast burrito with scrambled eggs, peppers, onions, and cheese (311 calories)
Lunch: Seafood soup with shrimp, fish, and vegetables (292 calories)
Dinner: Grilled chicken with roasted zucchini and brown rice (454 calories)
Snack: Plain Greek yogurt with sliced peaches (143 calories)

Day 7:
Breakfast: Cottage cheese with mixed berries and honey (215 calories)
Lunch: Grilled chicken with mixed greens and cherry tomatoes (284 calories)
Dinner: Baked tilapia with mixed veggies and quinoa (391 calories)
Snack: Sliced cucumber with hummus (92 calories)

All the meals mentioned above have been selected with precision and are balanced with protein, carbohydrates, and fats that will help you stay full for longer and keep your blood sugar levels in check.

Moreover, if you look closely, all the meals are nutrient-dense and include lots of fresh and wholesome ingredients, providing you with the necessary macro and micronutrients.

You may also find it helpful to use a basic calorie counting chart to keep yourself in check.

Essentially, this chart is just a table or spreadsheet where you can track the number of calories, macronutrients, and mealtimes for each of the foods you consume. You can create your chart with a pen and paper or a digital app to track it over time, for example, in your mobile phone.

Here's one I like to use:

Time	Date	Food	Calories
Total Daily Calories			

HOW TO READ AND UNDERSTAND FOOD LABELS

As you know now, knowing what to eat and what not to eat is crucial when it comes to managing your blood sugar levels. That easy when you're eating raw fruits and vegetables but what about when you are buying something off the shelves?

Understanding how to decode food labels is another important step in healthy eating to manage your type 2 diabetes. Here are some tips.

Start With the Serving Size

The serving size is displayed prominently on the top of the nutrition facts label.

Always start here because everything else on the label is based on this serving size. Most food products contain multiple servings, so it's essential to pay attention to how many servings you're consuming.

For example, if the serving size of a pack of cookies is two, but you eat the entire pack of ten, you need to increase the calories, carbs, and other nutrients listed on the label to accurately reflect your consumption.

Carb Content

When reading food labels, always check the total number of carbohydrates listed per serving size. It can be useful to compare the carb content of similar products to help you make the best choice. Look for products with fewer carbs, which can help you better manage your blood sugar levels.

Sugar and Sugar Substitutes

Many products contain added sugar, which can significantly affect your blood sugar levels. Pay attention to the total sugar content listed on the food label and avoid products with too much added sugar.

Always check the ingredient list for sugar substitutes like high fructose corn syrup, agave, or brown rice syrup. These substitutes may not spike your blood sugar as quickly as table sugar, but they can still affect your blood sugar levels.

Manufacturers sometimes use sneaky names for sugar, such as dextrose, sucrose, and maltodextrin. Watch out for other hidden ingredients too, such as trans fats, sodium, and artificial flavors and colors.

Alcohol's Effect on Glucose

Alcohol and glucose metabolism are closely linked. When you consume alcohol, your liver goes into overdrive to process it. This process slows down the release of glucose from the liver into the bloodstream, which can cause your blood sugar levels to drop. This drop can last for up to 24 hours after you've had your last drink.

As this impact on glucose control can put you at risk, it's crucial to maintain close blood glucose monitoring while drinking.

Another thing to factor in is the effect of mixers on glucose levels when drinking. If you add sugary drinks or mixers to your alcoholic drink, you're increasing your blood glucose levels with a similar effect on glucose metabolism. Mix alcohol with low or sugar-free options such as diet coke, sparkling water, or fresh citrus juices.

When planning to drink, remember that it can be a good idea to eat a meal containing complex carbohydrates like whole wheat bread, potatoes, peas, or beans. Eating these kinds of foods alongside your drink can help keep your blood sugar levels stable while you enjoy drinking.

It's advisable to monitor your blood glucose levels in the morning after a night of drinking, particularly before eating. Doing so will allow you to adjust your intake if you experience a reading that is beyond your target range.

The influence of alcohol on the glucose levels in the body can vary, so monitoring and taking slow and steady steps to adjust accordingly will be helpful in stabilizing blood sugar levels.

SMOKING AND DIABETES

Like alcohol, smoking and diabetes are two major health concerns that are also closely connected.

Smoking not only increases the risk of developing diabetes, but it can also make diabetes management more challenging. If you have type 2 diabetes, you need to take the time to understand the relationship between smoking and diabetes and take the necessary steps to quit smoking ASAP.

How Can Smoking Lead to Diabetes?

Several studies have shown that smoking results in insulin resistance, making it difficult for the body to use insulin effectively. As insulin is responsible for regulating blood sugar levels, impaired insulin function can lead to high blood sugar levels, a precursor to diabetes.

Smoking can also damage blood vessels and organs, leading to metabolic dysfunction that impairs glucose metabolism. And the list of problems doesn't end there—smoking can also increase cortisol levels, which causes high blood sugar levels.

Smoking if you have Diabetes

Smoking can make it challenging to manage diabetes and increase the complications associated with it. People with diabetes who smoke are more likely to develop cardiovascular disease, kidney disease, eye disease, and neuropathy.

Smoking narrows blood vessels, reducing blood flow to vital organs, and can cause nerve damage, which makes it difficult to feel foot injuries, infections, and wounds.

Smoking and Sleep

Smoking can also affect sleep quality, which impacts diabetes management (something I'll discuss in more detail in the next section).

People who smoke are more likely to snore and have sleep apnea. Sleep apnea can cause blood sugar levels to spike, leading to insulin resistance and making diabetes harder to manage.

Moreover, sleep-deprived individuals have impaired glucose metabolism and are more likely to make poor food choices that affect blood sugar levels.

Does Smoking Cause Diabetes?

Although smoking is not a direct cause of diabetes, it can increase the risk of developing type 2 diabetes.

Moreover, smoking can make it harder to control blood sugar levels once someone has diabetes. Smoking increases the risks of multiple health issues, and quitting smoking is an essential step toward optimal health.

Quitting Can Help

Quitting smoking is by far the most effective way to reduce the risks associated with smoking and diabetes. If you need help quitting, seek support from friends, family, or healthcare providers.

Nicotine replacement therapy, medication, and counseling can all help smokers quit smoking successfully and manage diabetes more effectively. Quitting can lower blood pressure, improve blood sugar levels, and reduce the risk of complications associated with diabetes.

SLEEP AND DIABETES

A good night's sleep doesn't just help you feel refreshed, it also helps you manage your diabetes. As someone living with diabetes, you need to understand how your sleeping habits can impact your blood sugar levels.

Sleep Can Both Raise and Lower Glucose Levels

Some individuals with diabetes may experience a rise in blood sugar levels during sleep, especially if the body releases stress hormones such as cortisol.

On the other hand, some individuals may experience a drop in blood sugar levels while sleeping, which is known as nocturnal hypoglycemia.

Therefore, it's essential to monitor your blood sugar levels regularly, especially before bedtime. You may want to consult with your doctor to adjust your medications, insulin, or diet to avoid experiencing sudden spikes or drops in your glucose levels.

Why Sleep Affects Blood Sugar

Researchers have found that lack of sleep or poor sleep quality can negatively impact insulin sensitivity, which is essential for your body to properly regulate blood sugar levels.

Moreover, a lack of sleep can increase stress hormones such as cortisol, which can lead to an increase in blood glucose levels. It's essential to aim for 7-8 hours of sleep per night to improve insulin sensitivity, avoid developing a resistant state, and lower your chances of developing type 2 diabetes complications.

Blood Sugar Levels May Also Impact Sleep Quality

On the flip side, elevated blood sugar levels can impact your sleep quality, too. Studies show that people with high blood sugar levels often experience low-quality sleep due to frequent urination, night sweats, and restless legs syndrome.

Maintaining good glycemic control is essential for achieving a restful and rejuvenating sleep. Be sure to manage your blood sugar levels during the day to enhance your chances of sleeping better at night.

Benefits of Good Quality Sleep

Getting optimal sleep every night is essential for people living with diabetes to achieve and maintain good health.

Adequate sleep has been linked to numerous benefits such as enhanced insulin sensitivity, improved blood sugar control, lowered risk of developing type 2 diabetes and its complications, reduced inflammation, lower stress levels, and enhanced mental and physical well-being.

To reap these benefits, aim for a healthy sleep schedule every night.

STRESS AND DIABETES

Stress is an inevitable part of our lives. Whether it's the stress of work, family, or finances, it takes a toll on our well-being. As a person with type 2 diabetes, you may be at a higher risk of experiencing stress-related complications. Stress can affect your blood sugar levels, making it harder to manage your diabetes.

Fortunately, there are ways to manage stress and lower your risk of developing diabetes-related complications. I won't go into too much detail here, since I'll tackle this topic in more depth later in the book.

However, for now, know that stress can affect your body in various ways. When you're stressed, your body responds by releasing stress hormones such as cortisol and adrenaline. These hormones cause your heart to beat faster, your blood pressure to rise, and your blood sugar levels to increase.

For people with diabetes, this can be particularly problematic. Chronic stress can make it harder to control your blood sugar levels, leading to long-term complications such as nerve damage and cardiovascular disease.

The first step in managing stress is to identify your triggers. What situations or events cause you the most stress? Once you've identified your triggers, come up with a plan to manage them. Some techniques that may work for you include practicing relaxation techniques such as deep breathing or meditation, exercising regularly, and talking to a trusted friend or family member.

Taking care of yourself is essential when it comes to managing stress and preventing diabetes-related complications. Make sure to get enough sleep, eat a healthy diet, and engage in activities that you enjoy. Self-care can also mean saying no to certain obligations or commitments if they're too stressful for you.

Of course, an essential part of self-care is making sure you eat a proper diet. Hopefully, you now have some good ideas of what that healthy diet might look like and ways you can start transitioning to a healthier eating plan today.

Don't beat yourself up if every meal or even every day of eating isn't perfect. There's room for enjoyment in a healthy diet if you strive toward healthy food choices 80% of the time, the remaining 20% can be left up to your own personal preference. Do your best, and you'll find that even the small changes start to add up to big results over time. Remember to keep sugar content in moderation but don't completely deprive yourself of your favorite things.

Diet is an obvious intervention for diabetes, but many people don't recognize the importance of the second most important diabetes treatment and lifestyle adjustment which is exercise.

Ready to get moving? Whether you're fond of jogging, swimming, Zumba, or powerlifting it's time to learn more about how exercise can be used to help you manage your type 2 diabetes.

BUILDING A COMMUNITY

"I May have diabetes, but diabetes does not have me."

— STAN B. BLACKARD

I'd like to ask you to take a moment to think about how you felt when you first received your diagnosis.

What emotions were running through you? Were you scared? Anxious? Overwhelmed? Did you ask yourself where you went wrong or if this was all your fault?

These are all common reactions to receiving a diagnosis of type 2 diabetes, and I've witnessed countless patients experience them. Suddenly being faced with a lifetime of glucose meters and insulin pumps is overwhelming, and it can make you feel very isolated – even though you know that many other people are living with the condition.

This is why I'm committed to supporting as many people as possible – and to help me do that, I'd like to ask you to get involved.

The good news is, doing so will barely make a dent in your schedule, and you don't even have to leave your chair. All I'd like you to do is leave a review.

By leaving a review of this book on Amazon, you'll help other people living with type 2 diabetes feel less alone and point them in the direction of the support and guidance they're looking for.

Simply by telling new readers how this book has helped you and what they'll find inside, you'll help me to provide support for more people.

Thank you so much for your help. We can't reverse that feeling someone gets when they first receive their diagnosis, but we can help them to take control going forward. Together, we can build a community.

Scan the QR code to leave a review!

6

EXERCISE AND PHYSICAL ACTIVITY FOR DIABETES MANAGEMENT

"I do not love to work out, but if I stick to exercising every day and put the right things in my mouth, then my diabetes just stays in check."

— HALLE BERRY

There's a saying that I like to live by on mornings where I'm finding it hard to get out of bed for my daily jog.

"A body in motion tends to stay in motion."

I've always found that after taking a few days away from my normal exercise routine, I have a really hard time getting back into it. It's very easy for a few days to turn into a few weeks, a few months, and before you know it, I'm back to being completely sedentary again.

The more I exercise, though, the easier it is for me to include it as part of my daily routine. It becomes second nature, just like brushing my teeth or taking a shower.

If you have diabetes, it's so important that exercise becomes part of your daily routine, too.

As the above quote from Haller Berry demonstrates, if you're able to prioritize your body by giving it what it needs via regular movement (and of course, the healthy diet I've already talked extensively about), you'll have a far easier time managing your diabetes than you would if you chose to live a more inactive lifestyle.

And if you're already active, diabetes shouldn't be viewed as an impediment to your active lifestyle. Just take the example of Peter Shaw, an avid kite surfer. He went out of his way to find an insulin pump with an on-board blood test meter that would allow him to continue to spend lots of time in the water (and in a wetsuit). Exercise should be part of your lifestyle, as someone with diabetes.

But why is that? And are all forms of exercise built alike in terms of their overall benefits? The answers to these questions might surprise you.

So, what are you waiting for? Lace up those sneakers and let's get a move on. It's time to learn about all the benefits associated with exercise for people with diabetes.

WHY YOU NEED TO GET ACTIVE AND START EXERCISING

When it comes to diabetes, even small amounts of exercise can make a big difference. For example, a 30-minute brisk walk after dinner can help regulate blood sugar levels and reduce the risk of complications. Exercise also helps to improve insulin sensitivity, which means your body can use insulin more efficiently.

Now that you understand the benefits of exercise, it's time to get started. If you are new to exercise, start slowly and gradually increase your activity level. Mix up your routine to keep it interesting and find activities you enjoy. Walking, swimming, dancing, and cycling are all low-impact exercises that are great for people with diabetes. Aim to be active for at least 30 minutes a day, most days of the week.

There are two types of exercise that are essential for people with diabetes: aerobic exercise and strength training.

Aerobic exercise includes things like walking, jogging, biking, or swimming which are activities you can do any day of the week. Strength training involves using weights or resistance bands to build muscle. Ideally, you should aim for two to three strength training sessions per week.

It's easy to make excuses for why you can't exercise.

For example, you may say you don't have enough time during the day or that you don't have access to a gym. But the truth is, you don't need a gym membership to be physically active.

Simple activities like taking the stairs instead of the elevator, walking your dog, or doing some light stretching while watching TV can all help to increase your daily activity. It's also important to schedule your exercise into your day and make it a priority. Treat your exercise time like an appointment that can't be missed.

When it comes to staying motivated, turning your excuses into solutions is key. If you have trouble finding a long block of time for exercise, try breaking it up into smaller increments throughout the day.

Maybe you can take a 10-minute walk during your lunch break or walk around your house during commercial breaks while watching TV.

Another plan is to buddy up with a friend or family member who also wants to be active. Having someone to exercise with can be more enjoyable and hold you accountable.

Remember to track your progress and celebrate your successes, no matter how small. This can help keep you motivated and remind you why you started in the first place.

DIABETES AND EXERCISE: WHEN TO MONITOR YOUR BLOOD SUGAR

It's important to keep in mind that your blood sugar levels can be impacted by movement, especially at first, if your body isn't quite used to it yet.

Below, I'll give you some general guidelines on how and when to check your blood sugar levels as part of your fitness routine.

Recommended Exercise Guidelines

It's essential to monitor your blood sugar levels before exercising, especially if you take insulin or other diabetes medications. This can help you determine whether you need to adjust your medication dosage or eat a snack to avoid hypoglycemia (low blood sugar).

If your blood sugar is too high, it's best to wait until it's back to a healthy range before beginning exercise.

You should also check your blood sugar levels every 30 minutes during exercise, especially if you're new to exercise, trying a new activity, or exercising for an extended period. This can help you determine whether you need to reduce the intensity of your workout, take a break, or eat a snack to avoid hypoglycemia.

If your blood sugar is too low, stop exercising, and eat a small snack or drink some juice to bring your levels back up.

And after exercise, checking your blood sugar levels can help you determine how your body responds to exercise and whether you need to make any adjustments to your diabetes management plan. If your blood sugar levels are too low, eat a snack or drink some juice to bring them back up. If your blood sugar levels are too high, it's essential to monitor them closely and possibly adjust your diabetes medication dosage or diet plan.

DIFFERENT TYPES OF EXERCISE AND HOW THEY AFFECT BLOOD SUGAR

Aerobic exercises such as brisk walking, cycling, and swimming can help your body use insulin efficiently and lower your blood sugar levels. During aerobic exercise, your heart rate increases, and your muscles use more glucose for energy.

This increases the number of insulin receptors your cells need to uptake insulin. This type of exercise is good for those with diabetes because it can help reduce the amount of medications or even insulin injections needed. Aim for 150 minutes of moderate-intensity aerobic activity per week and break this down into at least 30 minutes, 5 days a week.

Strength training exercises such as lifting weights, resistance band exercises and Pilates are also good for those with type 2 diabetes. Strength training can be an effective way to improve insulin sensitivity and decrease blood sugar levels.

If you can, you should perform these exercises at least two days a week, allowing 48 hours between workouts.

Aerobics and strength-training are the two most common "categories" of exercise, but there are a few other varieties to keep in mind as well.

One is HIIT. High-Intensity Interval Training is a type of exercise that involves short periods of intense activity followed by a short period of rest or a slower activity. This type of exercise has been shown to improve blood sugar control and lower A1C levels in those with type 2 diabetes. It can be challenging, so it's essential to listen to your body and consult with a healthcare professional before starting.

Flexibility training or stretching exercises such as yoga are good for maintaining mobility, stability, and balance. These exercises can improve blood glucose levels indirectly by reducing stress levels and boosting your metabolism. You can stretch for a few minutes every day or incorporate yoga classes into your exercise routine.

Finally, mind-body exercises such as tai chi and qigong are great for reducing stress levels and improving blood sugar levels. These types of exercises focus on meditation, deep breathing, and slow, flowing movements that can help decrease blood pressure and improve feelings of well-being.

SAFETY CONSIDERATIONS FOR EXERCISE WITH DIABETES

Exercise plays an essential role in the management of diabetes. However, exercise-induced hypoglycemia is one of the significant concerns people with diabetes face. Exercise can make it challenging to maintain blood glucose levels during and after physical activity.

In addition to regularly checking and monitoring your blood sugar levels, as mentioned earlier, there are some basic safety tips you'll want to follow.

For starters, you should always carry a source of glucose with you, such as candies, glucose tablets, or a sports drink. If you experience symptoms of hypoglycemia, you can consume these drinks to bring your blood glucose levels back to normal.

If you are new to exercising, it's recommended to start with low-intensity exercises and gradually increase the intensity levels. Sudden and drastic changes to your exercise routine can affect your blood glucose levels and can be a potential risk for hypoglycemia. Always consult with your doctor before starting any exercise routine.

Always keep a record of your workout routine, blood glucose levels, and any other relevant information. This helps you identify how different exercises affect your glucose levels. You can make the necessary adjustments to your diet, medication, and exercise routine to maintain healthy glucose levels.

Keeping yourself hydrated is also smart, especially when you are exercising. Dehydration can affect your glucose levels and lead to potential risks. Drink plenty of fluids before, during, and after exercise. Remember to always keep a water bottle with you during workouts.

IMPORTANCE OF INCORPORATING PHYSICAL ACTIVITY INTO YOUR DAILY LIFE

At this point, I hope you're convinced that the benefits of regular physical activity are numerous, particularly for people with type 2 diabetes. In addition to improving insulin sensitivity and glycemic control, suitable physical activity can reduce blood pressure, improve cholesterol levels, and increase cardiovascular health.

Moreover, regular exercise can benefit your mental health by reducing anxiety and depression levels, boosting mood, and improving sleep quality.

However, even with all the benefits that come with exercise, it can be difficult to get started or stay motivated.

Be patient with yourself and remember to consult your doctor before starting a new routine. By setting achievable goals and taking things one day at a time, you'll not only help to alleviate some of the symptoms of your type 2 diabetes, but you may be able to prevent further complications from taking hold.

Having covered these basic lifestyle adjustments as the first line treatments for managing diabetes, let's move on to ways you can prevent possible (and potentially major) complications that might come about because of diabetes.

7

MANAGING TYPE 2 DIABETES COMPLICATIONS

"Trying to manage diabetes is hard because if you don't, there are consequences you'll have to deal with later in life."

— BRYAN ADAMS

Living with type 2 diabetes can feel like a full-time job. It can be tough to deal with the balancing act of managing blood sugar levels while also preventing complications, but this is something that you've got to prioritize if you want to stay healthy and well.

It's not always the most fun. And it can be overwhelming!

But living with type 2 diabetes isn't just about avoiding and managing systems of the diabetes itself, but also preventing future complications. This chapter won't be the sunniest or the most cheerful, but it's important to understand potential outcomes of this disease if you want to avoid them.

Let's take a closer look at some of the most common complications of type 2 diabetes and how they can be avoided.

WHAT ARE THE RISKS OF UNCONTROLLED GLUCOSE COMPLICATIONS?

If you have type 2 diabetes, you already know that managing your blood sugar levels is imperative.

But did you know that uncontrolled blood sugar levels can lead to several serious complications? Don't panic just yet. With the right treatment and prevention strategies, you can keep these common complications at bay.

Awareness and education are key to helping you manage your diabetes and prevent future issues. If you take home anything from this book, let this be it!

I want to give you an overview of some common complications, not to scare you, but to keep you informed of potential risks so that you can take steps to actively avoid them.

Increased Risk of Heart Disease

One of the most significant problems associated with elevated blood glucose levels is an increased risk of heart disease. This is because high levels of glucose in the blood can damage the blood vessels and arteries, making it easier for plaque to build up and leading to the narrowing of the arteries.

Over time, this can reduce blood flow to your heart, leading to chest pain, heart attack, or stroke. It's essential to keep your blood glucose levels under control to reduce your risk of heart disease and other related problems.

Kidney Problems

When your blood sugar levels are uncontrolled, your kidneys must work overtime to filter out waste from your body. When your blood glucose levels are consistently high, it can lead to damage to the tiny blood vessels in your kidneys. This can lead to kidney damage or even kidney failure if left untreated.

To avoid this, make sure to control your blood sugar levels through a healthy diet, exercise, and medication as prescribed by your doctor. It's also important to keep an eye on your blood pressure and cholesterol levels, as high levels of these can also damage your kidneys.

Diabetes is the leading cause of kidney failure, so it's crucial to keep a close eye on your blood glucose levels to protect your kidneys and overall health. If you're experiencing symptoms such as increased urination, fatigue, or swelling in your legs and ankles, consult your doctor immediately.

Eye Problems

High blood glucose levels can also impact the small blood vessels in your eyes, leading to a variety of eye problems. These problems can include everything from minor changes in vision, to more complex issues such as glaucoma, cataracts, and diabetic retinopathy, and even permanent vision loss.

By keeping your blood glucose levels under control, and within a healthy range, you can help manage the progression of these issues and potentially even prevent them altogether.

It's also important to get regular eye exams from an optometrist or ophthalmologist. If you're experiencing symptoms such as eye pain, redness, or sudden changes in vision, seek medical attention right away.

Just look at the example of Rachael, a chiropractic office assistant and virtual assistant for the diabetes health coaching service Needles and Spoons.

Rachael has type 1 diabetes, so the story here is a bit different than the journey someone might experience with type 2 diabetes. Nevertheless, the potential risks and outcomes are the same.

Rachael was diagnosed with diabetes at the age of just four years old. She had managed the disease all her childhood and most of her adult life, until one day, when she was watching television with her husband, she noticed a spot in her vision. After having it checked out, she discovered she had bleeding in her retina. At the age of just 29 years old, she was legally blind.

The takeaway here is that it is so important to keep up with your eye appointments. Make sure your optometrist checks your vision and takes detailed photographs of your retinas. If you aren't happy with your eye care, get a new doctor. Diabetic retinopathy can happen to anyone, but with the right prevention and medical care, you can avoid or manage it should it happen to you.

Metabolic Syndrome

Metabolic syndrome is a group of conditions that increase your risk of heart disease, stroke, and diabetes. These conditions include increased waistline, high blood pressure, increased blood sugar, and obesity. Uncontrolled glucose levels exacerbate this risk by damaging your blood vessels and reducing insulin sensitivity. Symptoms include fatigue, pain, depressed mood, anxiety, and stress. Prevention and treatment strategies include controlling your glucose levels, managing your weight, and engaging in regular exercise.

Dementia

Studies have shown that people with type 2 diabetes are at a higher risk of developing dementia as they age. Dementia is a term given to a group of symptoms related to cognitive decline, such as memory loss and difficulty in communicating.

While the exact reasons for the link between diabetes and dementia are still unclear, researchers suggest that high glucose levels damage blood vessels in the brain, leading to cognitive problems such as memory loss, reduced ability to organize, confusion, disorientation, and changes in personality.

To minimize the risk of dementia, it's important to keep your glucose levels under control, exercise regularly, and maintain a healthy diet.

Sexual Dysfunction

Sexual health is also impacted by uncontrolled glucose levels. High glucose levels can lead to nerve and blood vessel damage, which can result in erectile dysfunction in men, and decreased sexual response and lubrication in women.

These sexual problems can seriously affect your quality of life and your relationship. Talking to your healthcare provider about these issues can help you get the appropriate treatment.

Neuropathic Pain

People with diabetes often experience neuropathic pain, which is a result of nerve damage. This commonly affects the feet and legs, but it can impact other areas of the body as well.

Uncontrolled glucose levels can worsen this pain, making it difficult to move around and perform daily activities.

Symptoms of neuropathy often include numbness, tingling, and even a sense of burning or pain. Neuropathy can also impact your ability to feel changes in temperature or pressure, which can lead to more serious problems, such as foot ulcers and infections.

Neuropathic pain can be a challenge to treat, but there are several interventions including various medications and complementary therapies that can alleviate the symptoms. Therapies and interventions include physical therapy, diabetic shoes or orthotics, TENS unit use, and acupuncture. Typical anti-inflammatory drugs and pain relief do not treat nerve pain and it is irreversible damage. The best way to treat neuropathic pain is to prevent it from happening. Anti-seizure drugs and some anti-depressants are used to help with neuropathic pain. Topical pain medications and supplements such as B vitamins, alpha lipoic acid, and acetyl-L-carnitine are often used to help with neuropathy.

Poor Wound Healing

One of the immediate and most obvious risks of uncontrolled glucose levels is poor wound healing. This presents as wounds that are difficult to close, where the skin has trouble reconnecting and closing over the wound. People with Type 2 diabetes are at an increased risk of developing cuts, bruises, and other injuries.

When blood glucose levels aren't adequately managed, the immune system is weakened, inhibiting the body's natural ability to heal. This can lead to more serious infections, a longer recovery time, and, in some cases, amputation.

Diabetic patients should see a podiatrist and have their feet checked regularly for poor healing ulcers and wounds. Wounds can occur anywhere but in patients with neuropathy they lose feeling in their feet and don't realize they have developed sores.

Immune Function Issues

As mentioned earlier, uncontrolled glucose levels also impact your immune function. When the body can't process glucose correctly, it can't produce enough energy for the cells, leading to decreased levels of white blood cells. This means that your body is more susceptible to infections and diseases.

Poor Circulation

High blood sugars can lead to a plaque buildup in your arteries. This restricts blood flow to various organs, which can cause systemic issues such as neuropathy, kidney disease, and heart disease. Poor circulation also affects the duration taken for a wound to heal, leading to more complications.

Trouble Breathing

While it's not widely known, Type 2 diabetes can increase the risk of lung diseases like asthma and chronic obstructive pulmonary disease (COPD). High blood sugar levels have been linked to reduced lung function, making breathing difficult, especially during and after exercise.

It's also possible that uncontrolled glucose levels can cause inflammation in the lungs, which can lead to these issues.

Increased Risk of Heart Disease

One of the most significant problems associated with elevated blood glucose levels is an increased risk of heart disease. This is because high levels of glucose in the blood can damage the blood vessels and arteries, making it easier for plaque to build up and leading to the narrowing of the arteries.

Over time, this can reduce blood flow to your heart, leading to chest pain, heart attack, or stroke. It's essential to keep your blood glucose levels under control to reduce your risk of heart disease and other related problems.

Cancer

People with Type 2 diabetes are at an increased risk of several types of cancer, including liver, pancreatic, and colon cancer. Although researchers aren't yet sure why this is the case, it's believed that elevated glucose levels might be a contributory factor.

As you can see, high blood glucose levels are no joke. They can lead to a variety of serious health problems that can significantly impact your quality of life. That's why it's so important to stay on top of your blood glucose levels and work with your healthcare team to manage your diabetes effectively.

Knowledge is Power

This last chapter may seem a bit bleak, and while it's not my goal to scare you or send you into a panic, I do think it's important to highlight some of the risks of type 2 diabetes. It's a serious condition, and as such, it's one you need to *take* seriously.

The good news is that there are plenty of steps you can take to manage your type 2 diabetes, some of which we've already covered in this book and involve basic lifestyle modifications.

And when those aren't enough, there's medication. Mainstream medicine is a beautiful thing and has brought us many ways to both treat and manage type 2 diabetes. Let us take a closer look at what some of these options are.

8

THE ROLE OF MEDICATIONS IN TYPE 2 DIABETES MANAGEMENT

"Laughter is the best medicine—unless you're diabetic, then insulin comes pretty high on the list."

— JASPER CARROTT

I promised a more lighthearted chapter, and here it is.

We all know that diabetes is no laughing matter. However, as something you must live with, it's important to have a good sense of humor, hence, the quote I included above. Make sure you have your medications under control before you start your standup comedy tour, please.

There are a few different types and classes of medications that can be used to treat type 2 diabetes and its symptoms. Obviously, lifestyle modifications are a huge part of managing disease, but medications also play an integral role.

In this chapter, I'd like to break those medications down a bit for you. Whether you've already been prescribed with one of them and are curious about how exactly it works or if you haven't yet talked to your doctor about which medications might be right for you it's my hope that this chapter can help clear things up for you.

Let's look, shall we?

TYPES OF MEDICATIONS FOR BLOOD SUGAR CONTROL

Managing blood sugar levels is crucial for people with type 2 diabetes. The good news is that there are different types of medications available to help in controlling blood sugar levels. However, the wide variety of options can leave you wondering which medication suits you best.

Some of the following information may be a review of what we covered earlier in this book, but I'm including it here again to make sure everything is crystal clear for you. If you have any questions, be sure to talk to your doctor for more information.

One more note before I dive into the nitty gritty of which options are available, all drugs do have the risk for side effects. Though most of these side effects are minor and are not life-threatening, it's important to be aware of them. I've detailed them below.

If you experience side effects with any of these drugs that are interfering with your quality of life, be sure to ask your doctor if there are alternative drugs that might be used in their place.

Insulin

If you've read through the earlier chapters, you'll already know that insulin is a hormone produced by the pancreas to regulate blood sugar levels. However, people with type 2 diabetes do not produce enough insulin, or their bodies have become resistant to insulin, requiring injections to regulate their blood sugar levels. There are various forms of insulin that cater to different needs.

Short-Acting Insulin

Short-acting insulin (also called regular insulin) is taken before meals to help control blood sugar spikes. This insulin works in about 30 minutes after injections, peaks in 2-3 hours, and lasts 3-6 hours. Examples include Human Regular (Humulin R, Novolin R).

Rapid-Acting Insulin

Rapid-acting insulin is taken before meals and begins working much faster than short-acting insulin. This insulin works about 15 minutes after injection and peaks in 1-2 hours, providing insulin coverage for 2-4 hours. Examples include insulin aspart (Fiasp, Novolog), insulin glulisine (Apidra) and insulin lispro (Admelog, Humalog, Lyumjev).

Intermediate-Acting Insulin

Intermediate-acting insulin takes longer to start working and lasts longer than rapid-acting insulin, making it a good option for overnight periods. This insulin takes effect 2-4 hours after injection, peaks in 4-12 hours, and is effective for 12-18 hours. Examples include NPH insulins (Humulin N, Novolin N, ReliOn).

Long-Acting Insulin

Long-acting insulin lasts for a full 24 hours and should be taken once a day. This insulin takes several hours to take effect and provides glucose lowering for 24 hours. Examples include Insulin degludec (Tresiba), detemir (Levemir), and glargine (Basaglar and Lantus).

Ultra Long-Acting Insulin

Ultra long-acting insulin reaches the blood stream in 6 hours, does not peak, and lasts 36 hours or longer. One example is insulin glargine U-300 (Toujeo).

Premixed (Combination) Insulins

Not everyone with diabetes requires insulin injections, however. For those who have lower daily insulin requirements, there are other options available, such as premixed (combination) insulins.

As the name suggests, these are a mixture of two different types of insulin that provide both a rapid and long-acting treatment in a single injection. This includes insulin 70/30, although you won't see these as often anymore.

Amylinomimetic Injectables

Amylinomimetic injectables, also referred to as amylinomimetic hormones, work differently than insulin. They work to suppress glucagon, a hormone that raises blood sugar levels, and thus lower blood sugar overall.

They are usually taken in combination with insulin injections and work to decrease the amount of insulin needed overall. One example is Symlin.

SGLT2 Inhibitor Drugs

These drugs are fairly new and are a class of medication used to help lower blood sugar levels in people with type 2 diabetes. How do they work?

SGLT2 inhibitors function by blocking the SGLT2 protein in the kidneys. This protein is responsible for reabsorbing glucose into the bloodstream from the kidneys. By blocking this protein, glucose is instead excreted through urine, leading to lower blood sugar levels.

Canagliflozin

Canagliflozin is sold under the brand name Invokana. Canagliflozin has been shown to lower A1C levels (a blood test that measures average blood sugar levels over a 3-month period) by 0.8-1.0%. Potential side effects include genital yeast infections and urinary tract infections.

Dapagliflozin

Dapagliflozin, or Farxiga, has been found to lower A1C levels by 0.6-0.7% and has the added bonus of potentially aiding in weight loss. However, like canagliflozin, urinary tract and genital infections are potential side effects.

Empagliflozin

Empagliflozin, or Jardiance, is another type of SGLT2 inhibitor. Compared to canagliflozin and dapagliflozin, empagliflozin has been found to have a greater impact on reducing the risk of heart disease in people with type 2 diabetes. Empagliflozin has also been shown to lower A1C levels by 0.6-0.7%.

Ertugliflozin

Finally, there's ertugliflozin, which is sold under the brand name Steglatro. Ertugliflozin has been found to lower A1C levels by 0.7-0.9% and can be taken alone or in combination with other diabetes medications. Like the other SGLT2 inhibitors, potential side effects include urinary tract and genital infections.

Biguanides

This drug works mainly by reducing the amount of glucose produced by your liver and helps improve insulin sensitivity. Metformin is the most commonly prescribed biguanide. It has a low risk of hypoglycemia, which makes it safe for use. It also helps with weight loss, making it an ideal option for people who need to lose weight while managing their diabetes.

Alpha-Glucosidase Inhibitors

Next up, we have alpha-glucosidase inhibitors. These drugs slow down the digestion of carbohydrates in the intestine, which reduces the amount of glucose released into the bloodstream after a meal.

Acarbose and miglitol are the two most used alpha-glucosidase inhibitors. These drugs, however, come with some gastrointestinal side effects, including bloating, diarrhea, and gas.

Dopamine-2 Agonists

Moving ahead, let's explore dopamine-2 agonists. These drugs work by increasing insulin sensitivity by affecting dopamine receptors found in the brain.

By doing so, they help reduce glucose production and help increase insulin sensitivity. Bromocriptine is the commonly used dopamine-2 agonist. It helps reduce fasting blood sugar levels without causing hypoglycemia or weight gain. An example is Cycloset (bromocriptine).

Dipeptidyl Peptidase-4 Inhibitors

These drugs work by blocking the action of the DPP-4 enzyme, which enhances insulin secretion. Sitagliptin and linagliptin are commonly used DPP-4 inhibitors. These drugs come with few side effects but must be used with caution in people with kidney disease. Examples include Januvia (sitagliptin), Onglyza (saxagliptin), Tradjenta (linagliptin), and Nesina (alogliptin).

Glucagon-Like Peptide-1 Receptor Agonists

This class of medication works by mimicking the body's natural hormone, GLP-1, which helps stimulate insulin secretion and lower glucose levels. GLP-1 agonists are available in both injectable and oral forms.

While they are effective in managing blood sugar levels, they can also come with some side effects such as nausea, vomiting, and diarrhea. Some examples of GLP-1 agonists include Byetta (twice daily) or weekly Bydureon (exenatide), Victoza (liraglutide), Trulicity (dulaglutide), Ozempic (semaglutide), and Rybelsus (oral semaglutide).

Meglitinides

Meglitinides are a type of medication that stimulates insulin release from the pancreas. They are taken orally before meals and work quickly to lower blood sugar levels. These medications can be effective for people who struggle with post-meal blood sugar spikes.

Examples of meglitinides include Prandin (repaglinide) and Starlix (nateglinide).

Sulfonylureas

Sulfonylureas have been around for over half a century and are still commonly used as a treatment for type 2 diabetes. They work by stimulating insulin secretion from the pancreas. Sulfonylureas are taken orally and are known to be very effective in lowering blood sugar levels.

However, they can also lead to weight gain and hypoglycemia. Common sulfonylureas include glipizide (Glucotrol), glimepiride (Amaryl), and glyburide (Diabeta).

Thiazolidinediones

TZDs are a type of medication that works by improving the body's sensitivity to insulin, which helps to control blood sugar levels. They are taken orally once a day and are effective in improving insulin resistance.

However, TZDs can also have some side effects such as fluid retention and an increased risk of fractures. Examples of

TZDs include pioglitazone (Actos) and rosiglitazone (Avandia).

WHICH OTHER MEDICATIONS CAN INTERFERE WITH DIABETES MEDICATIONS?

If you have type 2 diabetes and are taking medication to manage it, it's important to know that there are a few different medications that can interfere with your prescribed treatment.

And did you know that even certain over-the-counter medications can interfere with your diabetes medication? Yes, you read that right! These medications can affect your blood sugar levels and hinder your ability to control your diabetes.

Always talk to your doctor before taking *anything*, but here are some common medications that are known to interfere with diabetes treatments (I've included both OTC and prescription medications, for reference).

Pain Killers

Painkillers such as ibuprofen (Advil, Motrin) and codeine can raise blood glucose levels by blocking the effect of insulin. These medications are commonly used to manage pain and inflammation associated with arthritis, headaches, and menstrual cramps. It's essential to read the label carefully before taking these medications and consult your doctor if you're unsure about the potential risks.

Decongestants

Decongestants such as pseudoephedrine (Sudafed) and phenylephrine (found in many cough and cold products) are commonly used to treat cold and allergy symptoms. These medications can raise blood glucose levels by stimulating the liver to produce more glucose. It is recommended to avoid these medications altogether or take them under medical supervision.

Cough Syrups

Cough syrups containing sugar can significantly raise blood glucose levels. Moreover, coughing spells increase the body's demand for glucose, making it harder to manage blood sugar levels. It is advisable to opt for sugar-free cough syrups or those sweetened with alternative sweeteners. Look for cough syrups marked sugar free.

Anti-Diarrheal Medication

Anti-diarrheal medication such as loperamide (Imodium) can slow down the digestion process, leading to high blood sugar levels. Additionally, diarrhea can cause dehydration, making it harder to manage your blood sugar levels. If you need to take anti-diarrheal medication, make sure to monitor your blood sugar levels closely and drink plenty of fluids to stay hydrated.

Weight Loss Medication

Some weight loss medications, such as orlistat (Alli), can interfere with the body's ability to absorb fat-soluble vitamins and reduce insulin sensitivity. These effects can contribute to increased blood glucose levels and delay the management of diabetes.

Consult your doctor before taking any weight loss medication and shorten the duration of treatment to avoid adverse effects.

Steroids

Whether you're taking steroids (prednisone) for allergies, inflammation, or some other condition, they can interfere with diabetes medications by raising your blood sugar levels. So, if you're taking steroids, you may need to adjust your diabetes medications by talking to your doctor.

Beta Blockers

Beta blockers (metoprolol, propranolol, atenolol, carvedilol) are commonly used for high blood pressure and heart disease. However, they can also mask the symptoms of low blood sugar, which is a problem for people with diabetes who need to be able to recognize low blood sugar. If you're on beta blockers, talk to your doctor about how to monitor your blood sugar.

Diuretics

Diuretics (furosemide, torsemide, bumetanide) are used to treat conditions like high blood pressure and heart failure. However, they can also affect your blood sugar levels by increasing the amount of glucose your kidneys excrete. This can lead to high blood sugar levels. Again, talk to your doctor about adjusting your diabetes medication if you're taking diuretics.

Antipsychotics

Antipsychotic medications (risperidone, lurasidone, aripiprazole) are sometimes used to treat mental health conditions like schizophrenia and bipolar disorder. However, they can also cause weight gain, which can make it more difficult to manage diabetes. If you're taking antipsychotic medication, talk to your doctor about a plan to manage your weight.

Certain Antibiotics

Some antibiotics, like ciprofloxacin and levofloxacin, can lower blood sugar levels. This might be a good thing if you have high blood sugar, but if you're on other diabetes medications, it can be a problem. Always tell your doctor and pharmacist if you're taking these antibiotics and ask them if you need to adjust your diabetes medication.

BENEFITS AND RISKS OF MEDICATION THERAPY

First things first: Let's talk a little bit about the benefits and risks of medication therapy for type 2 diabetes. On the one hand, medications like metformin and insulin can help regulate blood sugar levels, reduce your risk of heart attack and stroke, and even improve symptoms of depression.

On the other hand, they can also cause side effects like nausea, dizziness, and gastrointestinal problems. If you're experiencing side effects from your medication, talk to your doctor. They may be able to adjust your dose or switch you to a different type of medication.

Another important thing to keep in mind is that different types of diabetes medications have different activation mechanisms.

For example, metformin works by reducing the amount of glucose produced by the liver and improving the body's sensitivity to insulin. Sulfonylureas, on the other hand, work by stimulating insulin production in the pancreas.

Depending on your individual needs and health history, your doctor may recommend one type of medication over another. If your medication isn't working as well as you'd like, it may be worth discussing alternative treatment options with your doctor.

WHAT TO DO IF YOUR DIABETES MEDICATION ISN'T WORKING

If you're concerned that your diabetes medication isn't working as well as it should be, don't hesitate to talk to your doctor. Your healthcare provider can run blood tests to assess your blood sugar levels and evaluate the effectiveness of your medication.

Depending on the results, they may recommend adjusting your dose, switching to a different medication, or offering additional support and resources to help you better manage your diabetes.

LIFESTYLE CHANGES VS MEDICATION: WHICH IS BEST?

Neither. Honestly, managing diabetes well involves an integrated approach that includes both lifestyle changes *and* medication.

Managing your diabetes isn't just about taking medication—it's also about making lifestyle changes that support your health and well-being.

Eating a nutritious diet, getting regular exercise, and managing stress can all play a role in keeping your blood sugar levels in check.

If you're struggling to adopt healthy behaviors, consider working with a registered dietitian, a personal trainer, or a mental health professional who can provide guidance and support.

THE COST OF INSULIN

If you ask somebody living with type 2 diabetes what the biggest challenges of managing their condition are, more than likely, the sky-high price of insulin will be at the top of that list. If you're one of those people, you've probably found yourself grappling with questions like: Why does insulin have to be so expensive? How can I afford to keep paying for it? And what happens if I can't?

The average price of insulin continues to rise, and while many drug manufacturers have capped their costs for consumers, it's still pricey—often more than $100 per month (with insurance).

The first thing you should do if you're struggling to keep up with the cost of insulin is talk to your doctor. While they might not be able to lower the price, they might be able to help you find affordable alternatives.

For example, there are insulin brands that are less expensive than others, and they may know which ones are covered by your insurance. There are also programs that offer financial assistance for people who can't afford insulin, and your doctor can help connect you with them.

You might also be surprised to learn that the cost of insulin can vary from one pharmacy to another. That's why it's a good idea to shop around and compare prices before filling your prescription if you are paying cash or using a discount card. Some pharmacies have their own discount cards developed to really help control costs.

Depending on your health insurance coverage, you might be able to switch to a high-deductible plan that has lower monthly premiums. Although you'll pay more out of pocket when you refill your insulin, you might end up saving money overall. Just be sure to talk with your doctor first to make sure that switching plans doesn't negatively affect your treatment.

WHY IT'S SO IMPORTANT TO STICK TO YOUR MEDICATION SCHEDULE

Managing diabetes is no walk in the park. It's a full-time job and takes a ton of discipline and focus. Having type 2 diabetes involves a lot of work, including regular visits to the endocrinologist, making lifestyle changes to better control your blood sugar levels, and of course, taking your prescribed medication on time, every time.

That might seem like tough work, but it is necessary to keep symptoms at bay and avoid further health complications. Your prescription drugs step in and control the amount of glucose in your bloodstream to maintain healthy levels.

Skipping doses can worsen or enhance your symptoms, depending on the situation, and it can throw your system off.

When your blood sugar levels are out of control, complications such as kidney disease, nerve damage, and vision problems can appear. Sticking to the prescribed medication is essential to prevent these severe complications from occurring.

As you know by now, from reading this book, the science of diabetes isn't cookie-cutter. The treatments and lifestyle changes that work for one person might not work as well for the next. While talking to your doctor about different medication options is always smart, it's also important to recognize that there are some strong mental and emotional factors that come into play when managing your type 2 diabetes.

If you don't recognize the ways in which diabetes affects your mental health, as well as your physical health, you can't be successful in managing it. In the next chapter, we'll take a closer look at some of the mental and emotional factors related to diabetes —and what you can do to manage those experiences, too.

9

MENTAL HEALTH AND EMOTIONAL WELL-BEING WITH DIABETES

"You can take hold of the situation. I feel great now. I live the right way. I wear fierce clothes. Everything I do now, I do it proud. I am a diabetic!"

— PATTI LABELLE

Living with type 2 diabetes can be challenging, but it doesn't have to be a dark cloud. Just like any other chronic illness, it presents a lifestyle change that requires focus and dedication. But it's important to remember that diabetes is not just about blood sugar levels and medication.

Managing your mental health and emotional well-being plays a vital role in your overall health and can help with managing your diabetes.

As Patti LaBelle said in her quote, you can take hold of the situation and live fiercely, even with diabetes. And part of that involves managing your mental health and emotional well-being.

In this next chapter, I'll give you some tips to help you navigate the emotional ups and downs of living with diabetes.

EMOTIONAL IMPACT OF A DIABETES DIAGNOSIS

I've noted several times that living with diabetes can be overwhelming. Suddenly, your life is filled with counting carbs, monitoring blood glucose levels, and worrying about potential complications.

All these responsibilities, on top of the emotional burden of a chronic illness, can be a lot to handle. It's important to acknowledge the emotional impact of a diabetes diagnosis and take steps to reduce stress and maintain your mental health.

How is Diabetes Linked to Emotion?

Managing diabetes can be frustrating, and it can make you feel as though your life is out of your hands. This lack of control can lead to feelings of anxiety and depression.

And what many people don't realize is that diabetes can affect your mood directly. It's not uncommon to experience mood swings because of fluctuating blood glucose levels. High blood sugar can cause irritability and fatigue, while low blood sugar can cause confusion, dizziness, and even seizures.

How Can I Reduce Stress in My Life?

Stress can cause blood sugar levels to rise, which can make managing diabetes more difficult. It's important to find healthy ways to cope with stress, such as exercise, meditation, or talking with a friend. It can also be helpful to limit your exposure to stressors in your life, such as negative news or toxic relationships.

Remember, self-care isn't selfish it's essential for maintaining your physical and emotional health.

Another way to reduce stress is to simplify your diabetes management routine. Talk to your healthcare provider about tools and resources that can make your life easier, such as a continuous glucose monitor or an insulin pump.

These devices can help take some of the burden off you and allow you to focus on living your life.

What Are the Symptoms of Depression?

It's not uncommon to experience feelings of sadness or anxiety after a diabetes diagnosis. However, if these feelings persist for more than a few weeks or begin to interfere with your daily life, you may be experiencing depression. Symptoms of depression can include:

- Persistent sadness or irritability
- Loss of interest in activities you once enjoyed
- Changes in appetite or weight
- Fatigue or loss of energy
- Difficulty sleeping or oversleeping
- Feelings of worthlessness or guilt

If you're experiencing any of these symptoms, it's important to speak with your healthcare provider. They can refer you to a mental health professional or provide other forms of support.

STRATEGIES FOR COPING WITH THE EMOTIONAL AND PSYCHOLOGICAL CHALLENGES OF DIABETES

Stress is a major contributor to high blood sugar levels, and diabetes management in and of itself can be very stressful, too.

Mindfulness and meditation can help you manage your stress levels and improve your mental wellbeing. Taking just a few minutes a day to focus on your breath and shift your attention away from your worries can have a huge impact on your diabetes management.

You may also want to consider setting some realistic goals. It's easy to get overwhelmed when you're trying to manage your diabetes. Setting unrealistic goals can make things even harder. Instead, focus on setting achievable goals and taking small steps towards them.

Celebrate your successes, no matter how small they may seem. Remember, any progress is progress.

Practicing gratitude can also help you shift your focus from what is going wrong to what is going right. It is easy to get bogged down by the challenges of living with diabetes, but taking time to recognize what you are grateful for can help you stay positive.

Start a gratitude journal, where you write down the things you are thankful for each day. Or take a few minutes each morning to reflect on what you are grateful for.

Finally, if you are finding it difficult to cope with the emotional and psychological challenges of type 2 diabetes, don't be afraid to seek professional help. Seeing a therapist or counselor can be incredibly helpful in managing stress and dealing with depression and anxiety. A healthcare professional can also help you to manage the physical aspects of your diabetes management.

IMPORTANCE OF SEEKING SUPPORT

Living with diabetes can feel isolating, but having a dedicated support system can help you stay motivated and positive. Talk to your friends and family about your challenges and let them help you.

Joining a diabetes support group or finding an online community can also be incredibly helpful. Surrounding yourself with people who understand what you are going through can make all the difference in the world.

Understanding Fact vs. Myth

There is a lot of misinformation out there about type 2 diabetes, which can make it difficult to manage. To start, it is important to separate the facts from the myths. This is where seeking support from healthcare professionals comes in.

A diabetes educator or a registered dietitian can help you understand the science behind managing your condition and separate the truth from the fiction. They can guide you in developing a healthy lifestyle that works for you, including meal planning, exercise, and medication management.

Support a Diabetes Charity or Organization

Another great way to seek support is to become involved with a diabetes charity or organization. These groups offer a wealth of information and resources for people living with diabetes, as well as opportunities to connect with others who are going through the same experiences.

You can participate in events, join support groups, and get involved in advocacy efforts to help raise awareness of the condition and its impact.

Not only will you be helping others, but you will also find encouragement and comfort in being part of a community that understands your experiences.

Find a Hobby that is Not Diabetes Related

Finding a hobby or activity that you love is a great way to relieve stress and take your mind off diabetes. This can be anything from gardening to painting to playing an instrument. The key is to find something that you enjoy and that isn't tied to your diabetes management.

Not only will you feel happier, but you'll also find that taking time for yourself can help you manage your diabetes better in the long run.

Open and Honest Communication

Seeking support from loved ones is crucial. They can offer emotional support, but it's important to communicate your needs effectively. Don't be afraid to let them know what you need from them, but also be an active listener in return.

Be willing to have open and honest conversations about how diabetes is affecting you and your relationship with them. By doing so, you can build a stronger support network that will help you manage your diabetes and feel more confident in your daily life.

THE ROLE OF STRESS AND ANXIETY IN BLOOD SUGAR CONTROL

When you're stressed or anxious, your body goes into fight-or-flight mode. This means that it releases hormones like cortisol, adrenaline, and glucagon that can increase your blood sugar levels. In people without diabetes, this isn't usually a problem—their bodies produce enough insulin to bring their blood sugar back down to normal levels.

But if you have type 2 diabetes, your body may not be able to produce enough insulin or use it effectively, which can lead to a dangerous spike in blood sugar.

It's not just acute stress that can impact your blood sugar, either. Chronic stress and anxiety can also take a toll on your diabetes management. When you're in a constant state of stress, your body is constantly releasing those blood sugar-raising hormones.

Over time, this can cause insulin resistance, meaning that your cells become less responsive to the insulin that your body does produce. This can lead to higher and higher blood sugar levels, making it more difficult to manage your diabetes.

So, what can you do to lower the impact of stress and anxiety on your blood sugar? The first step is recognizing when you're experiencing these emotions and taking steps to manage them. This could mean practicing relaxation techniques like deep breathing, meditation, or yoga, talking to a therapist or counselor, or even just taking a walk outside. Experiment with different strategies and find what works best for you.

Another important step is staying consistent with the other aspects of your diabetes management. When you're stressed or anxious, it can be easy to let things like exercise, healthy eating, and medication management fall by the wayside.

But sticking to your routine as much as possible can help keep your blood sugar levels steady and make it easier to manage the effects of stress and anxiety.

HOW TO PRIORITIZE SELF-CARE AND MENTAL HEALTH IN DIABETES MANAGEMENT

Remember that managing your diabetes and taking care of your mental health should be your top priority. Many people with diabetes tend to put others first, but it's important to remember that self-care comes first. Taking time for yourself is not selfish; instead, it helps you take better care of your loved ones and your health.

Make a list of things that you enjoy doing and set aside time to do them. It could be anything from reading a book, taking a walk, or even watching a movie. Any activity that brings you joy and reduces stress should be at the top of your list.

Managing diabetes is more than just taking medication and keeping your blood sugar levels under control. It's also about prioritizing your mental health and self-care. By practicing mindful eating, connecting with loved ones, prioritizing sleep, and taking other steps, you can make yourself a priority and keep your diabetes symptoms in check.

Managing your mental health and emotional well-being with diabetes takes time, effort, and dedication. But with the right strategies and support, it's possible to live a life of balance and confidence.

One key step in this process is to assess all the options for treating and managing your type 2 diabetes. This will empower you to advocate for the specific treatment you need. Plus, being well-informed helps you show your healthcare providers that you are actively taking charge of your health to the best of your ability.

Finally, don't be afraid to reach out for help if you need it. Managing diabetes is tough, and dealing with the additional stress and anxiety that comes with it can make it even tougher. But you don't have to go it alone. I hope that's something you now recognize after reading this chapter.

At the end of the day, remember to acknowledge and manage your emotions, take care of your physical health, connect with others who understand, shift your perspective, and celebrate your successes.

In the next chapter, I'll give you a little more insight on how you can use that "fierce" attitude to advocate for your own health and wellbeing. Let's take a look!

10

ADVOCATING FOR YOUR HEALTH WITH TYPE 2 DIABETES

"Empowering people with diabetes helps them make informed choices."

— MARY MACKINNON

Advocating for your health means taking an active role in your care. It means speaking up when you have questions or concerns, being prepared for doctors' visits, and staying informed about the latest research and treatments.

By advocating for your health, you can make sure that you receive the care and support you need to manage your condition effectively.

That said, being an advocate for yourself isn't always easy. You need to be able to speak up when you have concerns and to ask questions when you're curious—even if you think your questions might be "stupid."

As they told you in grade school, there's no such thing as a stupid question—and that's especially true when it comes to managing your type 2 diabetes.

Here are some tips to help you become your own best spokesperson and advocate.

WHY IT'S IMPORTANT TO BE AN ACTIVE PARTICIPANT IN HEALTHCARE DECISIONS

As a diabetic, you are your own advocate when it comes to your health. Being an active participant in your healthcare is crucial to ensure you receive the best possible treatment and care.

Not only will your healthcare providers better understand your unique medical history and needs, but you'll be able to make decisions based on your personal preferences and values while managing a chronic condition like diabetes.

Active participation also helps you build a collaborative relationship with your healthcare team, which leads to better care and improved outcomes.

WHAT TO CONSIDER WHEN COMMUNICATING WITH HEALTHCARE PROFESSIONALS

Effective communication with your healthcare team is key to ensuring that you receive the best care possible.

It is important to be open and honest about your medical history, symptoms, and concerns. You should also take the initiative to ask questions about your diabetes care and treatment and discuss your options.

Keep a list of any questions or concerns you have and bring them with you to appointments. This helps ensure that your healthcare provider addresses all your concerns and questions.

Bring any information from other providers such as labs, notes, and medication lists or changes. This helps communication between specialties, so everyone has an accurate picture of what is going on.

Remember, your healthcare team is there to help, and the more you communicate, the better they can assist you.

Questions to ask your healthcare provider.

Before starting any medication for diabetes, it's essential to have an open and thorough conversation with your healthcare provider to ensure the chosen medication is both safe and effective for your specific needs. To help guide your discussion, here are ten important questions you should consider asking your doctor or pharmacist:

1. What is the primary function of this medication?

Ask your healthcare provider about the intended purpose of the medication, how it works, and the expected benefits for your blood sugar management.

2. How and when should I take this medication?

Inquire about the appropriate dosage, timing, and whether the medication should be taken with or without food. This information is crucial to ensure proper absorption and effectiveness.

3. Can I take this medication with other drugs?

Discuss potential interactions with other medications you are currently taking and learn about any warning signs of adverse drug interactions.

4. Are there side effects or interactions with food or supplements?

Understand the potential side effects and any interactions with specific foods, beverages, or dietary supplements that could affect the medication's effectiveness or safety.

5. How long will it take before the medication begins to work?

Ask your healthcare provider about the expected time frame for the medication to start showing its effects on your diabetes.

6. How can I determine if the medication is working, and how frequently should I monitor my blood glucose?

Learn how to evaluate the effectiveness of your medication and the recommended frequency for blood sugar monitoring.

7. Are there any lifestyle changes I should make while taking this medication?

Discuss any recommended adjustments to your diet, exercise routine, or other lifestyle factors that may complement your high blood sugar treatment plan.

8. What precautions should I take while on this medication?

Understand any specific precautions you should be aware of while taking the medication, such as avoiding activities, foods, or beverages.

9. What should I do if I miss a dose or accidentally take too much medication?

Learn the appropriate steps to take in case you miss a dose or accidentally take more medication than prescribed.

10. When should I schedule a follow-up appointment to assess my blood pressure and evaluate the medication's effectiveness?

Determine the optimal time for a follow-up appointment to review your blood sugar levels and discuss the medication's effectiveness with your healthcare provider.

By asking these vital questions and staying informed about your medication and its potential interactions, you can better manage your high blood sugar and reduce the risk of complications. Remember, active involvement in your treatment plan and open communication with your healthcare team is key to achieving optimal blood sugar control and improving your overall health.

PATIENT RIGHTS AS A DIABETIC

It is essential to understand what your rights are, so you can exercise them, and take control of your health.

To start with, as a diabetic, you have the right to access medical care without discrimination. This means that doctors cannot refuse to see you or provide adequate care based on your diabetes. It also means that insurance companies cannot deny you coverage or charge you higher premiums because of your condition.

Diabetes management requires medication and regular testing, and you have the right to both. Your healthcare provider should help you find affordable medication and provide you with the necessary test supplies. If you are having trouble getting access to medication, seek out resources, like assistance programs or patient advocacy groups. Often manufacturers offer assistance programs or coupons for meters and sometimes testing supplies. Hospitals and clinics often have case workers that can help you get affordable supplies.

Also, you have the right to make decisions about your care, including which physician you see, what medications you take, and what treatments you undergo. Do not be afraid to speak up and ask questions during your appointments. Your healthcare providers should collaborate with you to develop a care plan that suits your needs.

THE ROLE OF TECHNOLOGY IN DIABETES MANAGEMENT

Living with diabetes can be tough. It takes a lot of hard work and dedication to maintain good blood sugar levels, and even then, it can still be a challenge. But here is some good news, technology is making diabetes management easier than ever before.

From blood glucose monitors to insulin pumps, there is a range of new devices available that can help you better control your blood sugar levels. And it is not just about the hardware—software and apps are also playing a role in diabetes management.

Let us start with blood glucose monitors. For many people with diabetes, monitoring blood sugar levels is a daily task. But traditional monitors can be painful and difficult to use. Today, there are better options available. Some monitors now offer pain-free testing, while others connect to an app so you can monitor your levels on your phone. There are even monitors that can automatically share your results with your doctor, giving them a better understanding of your overall health.

Another device that is gaining popularity is the smart insulin pen. This is a device that tracks your insulin doses and sends the information to your smartphone. It can also remind you when it is time for your next dose, helping you stay on top of your medication. For people who use insulin regularly, this could be a real game-changer.

Then there are insulin pumps. These devices make it easier to manage insulin therapy, as they deliver insulin automatically throughout the day. They can also be adjusted to match your activity levels and food intake, giving you more control over your blood sugar levels.

And like many other devices, they can be used in conjunction with an app to help you track your progress.

Technology is not just about hardware, though. There are also apps and software that can help with diabetes management.

For example, there are apps that can track what you eat and suggest healthy alternatives, helping you make better food choices. Others can remind you to take medication, monitor your blood glucose levels, or even offer support from other people with diabetes.

SELF-ADVOCACY FOR BETTER HEALTH OUTCOMES

Self-advocacy is also important when it comes to diabetes management. This means taking an active role in your own health and making sure you have the tools and resources you need to manage your condition. Technology can help with this, but it's important to be informed and to understand what's available.

Self-advocacy in a healthcare setting refers to the practice of patients or individuals taking an active and informed role in advocating for their own healthcare needs, preferences, and rights. It involves asserting one's interests, asking questions, and making decisions regarding their medical care, treatment options, and overall well-being. Self-advocacy is essential in empowering patients to:

1. Communicate Effectively: Express their concerns, symptoms, and medical history clearly to healthcare providers, ensuring accurate and comprehensive information is available for diagnosis and treatment.

2. Make Informed Decisions: Gather information about their medical condition, treatment options, potential risks, and benefits, enabling them to make informed decisions in collaboration with healthcare professionals.
3. Ask Questions: Seek clarification, ask questions, and request additional information about their diagnosis, treatment plan, and medications to ensure they understand and are comfortable with the proposed care.
4. Assert Preferences: Share their preferences and values regarding treatment approaches, pain management, and end-of-life care, allowing healthcare providers to tailor care to individual needs.
5. Advocate for Rights: Be aware of their legal and ethical rights as patients, including the right to informed consent, confidentiality, and access to medical records, and assert these rights when necessary.
6. Monitor Care: Keep track of their healthcare journey, including appointments, medications, and symptoms, to help identify any issues or discrepancies in their care.
7. Seek Second Opinions: If uncertain or dissatisfied with a diagnosis or treatment plan, patients can seek second opinions from other healthcare professionals to ensure the best possible care.

8. Address Concerns: Speak up if they experience any discomfort, side effects, or complications related to their treatment, ensuring timely interventions and adjustments.
9. Collaborate with Care Team: Work collaboratively with healthcare providers, nurses, and other members of the care team to achieve the best possible health outcomes.

Overall, self-advocacy in healthcare empowers individuals to actively participate in their healthcare decision-making process, promote their own well-being, and ensure that their medical care aligns with their values and preferences. It is particularly important in today's patient-centered healthcare systems, where shared decision-making and patient engagement are valued practices.

SPECIAL CONSIDERATIONS FOR DIABETES MANAGEMENT

Diabetes management differs depending on the demographic. Here are a few general guidelines for diabetes management across age groups.

Children

Managing diabetes in children can be challenging because they may not fully understand the disease and its impact on their daily lives. Plus, children often have difficulty adhering to strict diet and medication schedules.

As a result, caretakers must be particularly vigilant about monitoring blood sugar levels and ensuring children with diabetes receive appropriate support and education.

Adolescents

Adolescence is a time of significant physical and emotional changes, which can make diabetes management even more challenging. Adolescents with diabetes often struggle with self-care and maintaining healthy habits amidst peer pressure and other distractions.

One way to engage adolescents with diabetes in their care is to incorporate technology into their self-management routine.

For example, some teens may benefit from using diabetes management apps and wearable devices to track their blood sugar levels, physical activity, and medication adherence.

Elderly

Diabetes management in the elderly is often complicated by other health conditions and medications, which can interfere with blood sugar control. In addition, elderly patients may have difficulty adhering to strict dietary and exercise guidelines due to decreased mobility and cognitive function.

One way to support elderly patients with diabetes is to establish a strong care team that includes family members, healthcare providers, and pharmacists. It's also essential to customize treatment plans based on individual needs and preferences.

Because many elderly patients with diabetes have had the condition for many years, it's also important to recognize that your treatment and management of diabetes might change as you age.

Just take the example of Bob Krause, who died at the age of 90 due to complications unrelated to diabetes. Bob spent more than 85 years of his life with diabetes. He went down in history as the first American to live with diabetes for 85 years, and he witnessed remarkable changes as treatments for diabetes evolve over time.

Bob outlived the life expectancy of a normal healthy person born in 1921. -While he always knew he had to deal with his diabetes, he also recognized that it's just a part of his life and it doesn't need to control his life.

Perspective is everything, Bob is excellent proof of this.

PAY IT FORWARD

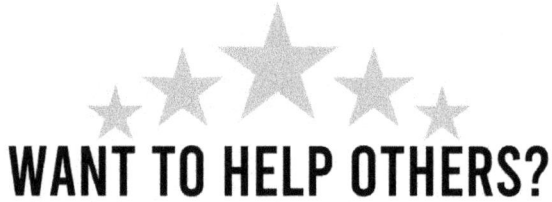

WANT TO HELP OTHERS?

As we've said, knowledge is power… and this is your chance to spread it to help others.

Simply by sharing your honest opinion of this book and a little about your own experience, you'll show new readers that they're not alone and there's guidance out there to help them take control.

If you found this book valuable and insightful, I would greatly appreciate it if you could take a moment to leave a review. Thank you for your support and sharing your thoughts!

Scan the QR code to leave a review!

Follow Dr. Ashley Sullivan, PharmD on Facebook and on her website ashleysullivanonline.com

CONCLUSION

Perspective is everything. That's something I said in the last chapter, and it's something I've reiterated continuously throughout this book.

While type 2 diabetes isn't necessarily something that's "fun" or "cool" to live with, the reality is that you can't change the diagnosis. The only thing you can change is your mindset.

Managing type 2 diabetes can be a daunting task, but it doesn't have to be. Often, we view diabetes as an enemy, and the thought of having to control what we eat, constantly monitor our blood sugar levels, and take medication can take a toll on us physically and mentally.

But what if we shift our perspective and look at it as a chance to take charge of our health?

Through the right mindset and perspective, we can turn what may seem like a burden into an opportunity to improve our overall well-being.

While it may be overwhelming to think about all the things that you cannot eat or do as a person living with type 2 diabetes, it's essential to focus on what you can control.

Take time to plan and prepare meals that are healthy and enjoyable at the same time. Engage in physical activities that bring you joy, and do not be afraid to try new things. Every person is different, and so is their experience with managing type 2 diabetes. Focus on finding what works best for you and incorporating it into your lifestyle.

Knowledge is power, and when it comes to managing type 2 diabetes, understanding the condition is crucial. Educate yourself on what type 2 diabetes is, the medication you are taking, and how to monitor your blood sugar levels.

The more you know, the more equipped you will be to make informed decisions and manage the condition effectively.

Hopefully, you now know the skills, techniques, and basic information you need to feel as though you can take charge of your type 2 diabetes. We have covered all the basics in this book so that you can control every aspect of your type 2 diabetes, including your:

- Mental health and emotional wellbeing
- Suitable lifestyle modifications

- Medications and the ability to adhere to them as prescribed
- Accountability, adherence, and self-advocacy for your own health

When we change the way we think about and view things, we empower ourselves to make better decisions and take control of our health.

Just take the example of Nan Hilton.

Nan was diagnosed with type 2 diabetes in 2006 at just 23 years old.

She took medications and insulin for years. When she became pregnant in 2010, she knew something needed to change. Her pregnancy was considered high-risk due to her diabetes, and during her pregnancy, she developed severe diabetic retinopathy that caused vision loss and required complicated, invasive surgery.

Her life changed dramatically due to her diabetes, to a debilitating point. After giving birth, she knew it was time for a major overhaul.

Nan made some basic lifestyle modifications (such as incorporating aerobic activity and changing her diet) that resulted in a 90-pound weight loss. Today, Nan no longer relies on diabetes medications. She leans on her family for support and relies on them to continue to provide her with the motivation she needs to stay on track.

You can do this, too.

Always remember, you are not alone. Millions of people are managing their type 2 diabetes and thriving. And with the right tools and support, you can too.

It has been a pleasure to walk you through everything you need to know about type 2 diabetes. I am hoping that this book has given you the confidence you need to take back control of your health and well-being.

If you enjoyed this book, please leave me a review. This will help other people like yourself find the book and access the information *they* need to take charge of their type 2 diabetes, too. As I have said repeatedly, knowledge is power. So please take the time to pay it forward and help others access this knowledge, too.

As Dale Evans famously said, "Life is not over because you have diabetes. Make the most of what you have."

Hopefully, this book has given you everything you need to move forward—and to live a healthy, prosperous life with type 2 diabetes.

GLOSSARY

Adiposity- body fat

Anabolic steroids- synthetic (man-made) versions of testosterone

Blood lipid levels- a panel of blood tests used to find abnormalities in lipids such as cholesterol and triglycerides

Blood Sugar- the concentration of glucose in the blood

Cataracts- a medical condition in which the lens of the eye becomes progressively opaque resulting in blurred vision

Cholesterol- a compound found in cell membranes and precursor to steroid compounds

Cognitive Function- brain functions (attention, memory, and processing speed)

Cortisol- A steroid hormone that your adrenal glands produce and release

Diabetic coma- severely high or low glucose levels can cause unresponsiveness

Emaciation- extreme loss of muscle and fat under the skin from malnutrition

Epigenetic- the study of how your behaviors and environment can cause changes that affect the way your genes work

Glaucoma- nerve damage in the eye from high eye pressure causing blindness

Glucagon- a hormone formed in the pancreas which promotes the breakdown of glycogen to glucose in the liver

Glucose- a simple sugar which is an important energy source and a component in carbohydrates

Glucose Meters- a device for measuring the concentration of glucose in the blood

Glycemic control- a medical term referring to the typical levels of blood sugar (glucose) in a person with diabetes mellitus.

Glycemic Index- a system that ranks foods on a scale from 1 to 100 based on their effect on blood sugar levels

HbA1c (A1c)- Hemoglobin A1C measures the amount of blood sugar (glucose) attached to your hemoglobin.

HDL- high-density lipoprotein is a type of cholesterol, sometimes called "good" cholesterol, which absorbs cholesterol in the blood and carries it back to the liver

Hyperglycemia- an excess of glucose in the bloodstream

Hypoglycemia- deficiency of glucose in the bloodstream

Insulin- a hormone produced in the pancreas which regulates the amount of glucose in the blood

Insulin Pump- An insulin pump is a medical device used for the administration of insulin in the treatment of diabetes

Insulin Resistance- an impaired response of the body to insulin resulting in elevated levels of glucose in the blood

Ketoacidosis- "Diabetic ketoacidosis" is a serious complication where the body produces excess blood acids (ketones)

Ketones- an organic compound that the liver produces when it breaks down fats

Metabolic Dysfunction- when something is wrong with the body's metabolism

Metabolic Syndrome- multiple abnormalities associated with the development of cardiovascular disease and type 2 diabetes

Net carbs- the total amount of fully digestible carbohydrates contained within a product or meal

Neuropathy- disease or dysfunction of one or more peripheral nerves typically causing numbness and weakness

Nocturnal Hypoglycemia- low blood sugar levels at night in a person who has diabetes

Obesity- the state or condition of being very fat or overweight

Prediabetes- impaired glucose tolerance

Retinopathy- a complication of diabetes that affects the eyes damaging blood vessels and leading to vision loss

Steroids- organic compounds in the body that makeup hormones

Triglycerides- the main constituents of natural fats and oils, high concentrations in the blood indicate an elevated risk of stroke

REFERENCES

Alcohol and diabetes. (n.d.). ADA. https://diabetes.org/healthy-living/medication-treatments/alcohol-diabetes

Are there any safety considerations for people with diabetes when they exercise? (n.d.). ViMax Media. Retrieved June 15, 2023, from http://erlr.org/generic/articles/diabetic-smart/are-there-any-safety-considerations-for-people-with-diabetes-when-they-exercise/

Assid, P. (2021). Diabetes and shortness of breath: What's the cause? *Verywell Health*. https://www.verywellhealth.com/diabetes-and-shortness-of-breath-5114863

Blood glucose. (n.d.). MedlinePlus. https://medlineplus.gov/bloodsugar.html

Blood glucose and insulin at work. (n.d.). ADA. https://diabetes.org/tools-support/diabetes-prevention/high-blood-sugar

Blood sugar testing: Why, when, and how. (2022). Mayo Clinic. https://www.mayoclinic.org/diseases-conditions/diabetes/in-depth/blood-sugar/art-20046628

BNF is only available in the UK. (n.d.). NICE. https://bnf.nice.org.uk/treatment-summaries/hypoglycaemia/

Budson, A. E. (2021). What's the relationship between diabetes and dementia? *Harvard Health*. https://www.health.harvard.edu/blog/whats-the-relationship-between-diabetes-and-dementia-202107122546

Callahan, A. (2018). 7 medications that may affect blood sugar control in diabetes. *EverydayHealth*. https://www.everydayhealth.com/type-2-diabetes/treatment/medications-may-affect-blood-sugar-control-diabetes/

Carbohydrates: How carbs fit into a healthy diet. (2022). Mayo Clinic. https://www.mayoclinic.org/healthy-lifestyle/nutrition-and-healthy-eating/in-depth/carbohydrates/art-20045705

Carbohydrates, proteins, fats, and blood sugar. (n.d.). HealthLink BC. https://www.healthlinkbc.ca/healthy-eating-physical-activity/food-and-nutrition/nutrients/carbohydrate-proteins-fats-and-blood

Care, D. (2018). 10 tips for effective communication with your doctor.

Diabetes Care Community. https://www.diabetescarecommunity.ca/living-well-with-diabetes-articles/10-tips-for-effective-communication-with-your-doctor/

CDC. (2018). All about your A1C. *Centers for Disease Control and Prevention.* https://www.cdc.gov/diabetes/managing/managing-blood-sugar/a1c.html

CDC. (2021). Make the connection. *Centers for Disease Control and Prevention.* https://www.cdc.gov/diabetes/managing/diabetes-kidney-disease.html

CDC. (2022a). Diabetes symptoms. *Centers for Disease Control and Prevention.* https://www.cdc.gov/diabetes/basics/symptoms.html

CDC. (2022b). Diabetes risk factors. *Centers for Disease Control and Prevention.* https://www.cdc.gov/diabetes/basics/risk-factors.html

CDC. (2022c). 10 tips for coping with diabetes distress. *Centers for Disease Control and Prevention.* https://www.cdc.gov/diabetes/managing/diabetes-distress/ten-tips-coping-diabetes-distress.html

CDC. (2022d). Sleep for a good cause. *Centers for Disease Control and Prevention.* https://www.cdc.gov/diabetes/library/features/diabetes-sleep.html

CDC. (2022e). What causes type 2 diabetes. *Centers for Disease Control and Prevention.* https://www.cdc.gov/diabetes/library/features/diabetes-causes.html

CDC. (2023a). Meal planning. *Centers for Disease Control and Prevention.* https://www.cdc.gov/diabetes/managing/eat-well/meal-plan-method.html

CDC. (2023b). Diabetes and mental health. *Centers for Disease Control and Prevention.* https://www.cdc.gov/diabetes/managing/mental-health.html

Chapple, Bridget. (n.d.). Stress and diabetes. *Diabetes UK.* https://www.diabetes.org.uk/guide-to-diabetes/emotions/stress

Cervoni, B. (2021). Are you more likely to get diabetes if it runs in your family? *Verywell Health.* https://www.verywellhealth.com/is-diabetes-genetic-5112506

Cherney, K. (2018). A complete list of diabetes medications. *Healthline Media.* https://www.healthline.com/health/diabetes/medications-list#type-1-diabetes

Chesak, J. (2020). What does insulin cost and what's behind the skyrocketing prices? *Verywell Health.* https://www.verywellhealth.com/insulin-prices-how-much-does-insulin-cost-and-why-5081872

Cervoni, Barbie. (2023). Could your diabetes medication stop working? *Verywell Health.* https://www.verywellhealth.com/diabetes-medication-not-working-6822997

Dening, J. (2022). What's the connection between diabetes and wound healing? *Healthline Media.* https://www.healthline.com/health/diabetes/diabetes-and-wound-healing

Devices & technology. (n.d.). ADA. https://diabetes.org/tools-support/devices-technology

Diabetes success stories. (2018). UMass Chan Medical School. https://www.umassmed.edu/dcoe/diabetes-care/success-stories/

Diabetes: 12 warning signs that appear on your skin. (n.d.). https://www.aad.org/public/diseases/a-z/diabetes-warning-signs

Diabetes and alcohol. (n.d.). WebMD. https://www.webmd.com/diabetes/guide/drinking-alcohol

Diabetes and blood sugar testing. (n.d.). WebMD. https://www.webmd.com/diabetes/home-blood-glucose-testing

Diabetes and cancer. (n.d.). ADA. https://diabetes.org/tools-support/diabetes-prevention/diabetes-and-cancer

Diabetes and dementia risk: Another good reason to keep blood sugar in check. (2021). Heart.org. https://www.heart.org/en/news/2021/07/21/diabetes-and-dementia-risk-another-good-reason-to-keep-blood-sugar-in-check

Diabetes and dietary supplements. (n.d.-). WebMD. https://www.webmd.com/diabetes/diabetes-dietary-supplements

Diabetes and dietary supplements. (n.d.). NCCIH. https://www.nccih.nih.gov/health/diabetes-and-dietary-supplements

Diabetes and exercise–Diabetes Stories. (n.d.). Diabetes Stories.https://diabetesstories.com/category/diabetes-and-exercise/

Diabetes and exercise: When to monitor your blood sugar. (2022). Mayo Clinic. https://www.mayoclinic.org/diseases-conditions/diabetes/in-depth/diabetes-and-exercise/art-20045697

Diabetes and Family History: How Much Risk is Genetic? (n.d.). YourDiabetesInfo.Org. https://yourdiabetesinfo.org/familyhistory/

Diabetes care and the adolescent population: Navigating the transition of roles and

responsibilities. (2022). NIDDK - National Institute of Diabetes and Digestive and Kidney Diseases. https://www.niddk.nih.gov/health-information/professionals/diabetes-discoveries-practice/managing-diabetes-transition

Diabetes diet: Create your healthy-eating plan. (2023). Mayo Clinic. https://www.mayoclinic.org/diseases-conditions/diabetes/in-depth/diabetes-diet/art-20044295

Diabetes management: How lifestyle, daily routine affects blood sugar. (2022). Mayo Clinic. https://www.mayoclinic.org/diseases-conditions/diabetes/in-depth/diabetes-management/art-20047963

Diabetes risk factors. (2018). Www.Heart.Org. https://www.heart.org/en/health-topics/diabetes/understand-your-risk-for-diabetes

Diabetes statistics. (2023). NIDDK: National Institute of Diabetes and Digestive and Kidney Diseases. https://www.niddk.nih.gov/health-information/health-statistics/diabetes-statistics

Diabetes: Stress & depression. Cleveland Clinic. (n.d.). https://my.clevelandclinic.org/health/articles/14891-diabetes-stress--depression

Diabetes treatment: Medications for type 2 diabetes. (2022). Mayo Clinic. https://www.mayoclinic.org/diseases-conditions/type-2-diabetes/in-depth/diabetes-treatment/art-20051004

Diabetes: What you need to know as you age. (2023). Johns Hopkins Medicine. https://www.hopkinsmedicine.org/health/conditions-and-diseases/diabetes/diabetes-what-you-need-to-know-as-you-age

Diabetic calorie counting chart. (2017). Diabetestalk.Net. https://diabetestalk.net/blood-sugar/diabetic-calorie-counting-chart

Diabetic nephropathy (kidney disease)— Symptoms and causes. (2021). Mayo Clinic. https://www.mayoclinic.org/diseases-conditions/diabetic-nephropathy/symptoms-causes/syc-20354556

Diabetic neuropathy. (2020). Johns Hopkins Medicine. https://www.hopkinsmedicine.org/health/conditions-and-diseases/diabetes/diabetic-neuropathy-nerve-problems

Diabetic neuropathy— Symptoms and causes. (2022). Mayo Clinic. https://www.mayoclinic.org/diseases-conditions/diabetic-neuropathy/symptoms-causes/syc-20371580

Diabetic retinopathy—Symptoms and causes. (2023). Mayo Clinic. https://www.mayoclinic.org/diseases-conditions/diabetic-retinopathy/symptoms-causes/syc-20371611

Do I need to change my type 2 diabetes medication? (n.d.). WebMD. https://www.webmd.com/diabetes/change-type-2-diabetes-meds

Drugs vs. lifestyle for preventing diabetes. (2016). NutritionFacts.Org. https://nutritionfacts.org/2016/03/08/drugs-vs-lifestyle-for-preventing-diabetes/

Doskicz, J. (2018). These 9 drugs may raise your blood sugar. *GoodRx.* https://www.goodrx.com/conditions/diabetes/drugs-that-raise-blood-sugar

Erectile dysfunction and diabetes: Take control today. (2023). Mayo Clinic. https://www.mayoclinic.org/diseases-conditions/erectile-dysfunction/in-depth/erectile-dysfunction/art-20043927

Exercise and diabetes. (2019). The Johns Hopkins Patient Guide to Diabetes. https://hopkinsdiabetesinfo.org/exercise-and-diabetes/

Exercise can raise blood glucose (blood sugar). (n.d.). ADA. https://diabetes.org/healthy-living/fitness/why-does-exercise-sometimes-raise-blood-sugar

Exercising safely with diabetes. (2016). Harvard Health. https://www.health.harvard.edu/diseases-and-conditions/exercising-safely-with-diabetes

Fallabel, C. (2022). Know your hospital rights as a person with diabetes. *Diabetes Daily.* https://www.diabetesdaily.com/learn-about-diabetes/living-with-diabetes/navigating-the-healthcare-system-with-diabetes/know-your-hospital-rights-as-a-person-with-diabetes/

Family health history and diabetes. (2023). CDC. https://www.cdc.gov/genomics/famhistory/famhist_diabetes.htm

The link between diabetes and sexual dysfunction. (2020). Cleveland Clinic. https://health.clevelandclinic.org/the-link-between-diabetes-and-sexual-dysfunction/

Fletcher, J. (2019). A list of healthier foods for people with diabetes, and foods to limit or avoid. *Medical News Today.* https://www.medicalnewstoday.com/articles/317355

Gasnick, K. (2023). Addressing sedentary lifestyle with type 2 diabetes. *Verywell Health.* https://www.verywellhealth.com/addressing-sedentary-lifestyle-with-type-2-diabetes-6606484

Genetics of diabetes. (n.d.). ADA. https://diabetes.org/diabetes/genetics-diabetes

Glucose Metabolism—An overview. (n.d.). ScienceDirect Topics. https://www.sciencedirect.com/topics/medicine-and-dentistry/glucose-metabolism

Gourmet, D. (2017). Best diabetes websites – hand-picked list. *Diabetic*

Gourmet Magazine. https://diabeticgourmet.com/articles/best-diabetes-websites-hand-picked-list

Gray, A., & Threlkeld, R. J. (2019). Nutritional recommendations for individuals with diabetes. *NCBI Bookshelf*. https://www.ncbi.nlm.nih.gov/books/NBK279012/

Gunnars, K. (2021). Carbohydrates: Whole vs. refined—here's the difference. *Healthline Media*. https://www.healthline.com/nutrition/good-carbs-bad-carbs

Halvorson, M., Yasuda, P., Carpenter, S., & Kaiserman, K. (2005). Unique challenges for pediatric patients with diabetes. *Diabetes Spectrum, 18*(3), 167–173. https://doi.org/10.2337/diaspect.18.3.167

Hazlegreaves, S. (2019). Technology and diabetes: How can innovation address the mounting challenge? *Open Access Government*. https://www.openaccessgovernment.org/technology-diabetes-challenge/59130/

Health checks for people with diabetes. (n.d.). ADA. https://diabetes.org/diabetes/newly-diagnosed/health-checks-people-with-diabetes

Herndon, J. (2021). What to know about steroid-induced diabetes. *Healthline Media*. https://www.healthline.com/health/diabetes/steroid-induced-diabetes

Hoskins, M. (2022). Helping you understand 'normal' blood sugar levels. *Healthline Media*. https://www.healthline.com/health/diabetes/normal-blood-sugar-level#target-glucose-goals

How can you support someone with diabetes in a nonjudgmental way? (2021b). *Verywell Health*. https://www.verywellhealth.com/supporting-someone-with-diabetes-5206667

How diabetes affects employment and daily work. (2019). dQ&A. https://d-qa.com/how-diabetes-affects-employment-and-daily-work/

How secreted insulin works in your body. (n.d.). WebMD. https://www.webmd.com/diabetes/insulin-explained

How sleep affects blood sugar. (n.d.). WebMD. https://www.webmd.com/diabetes/sleep-affects-blood-sugar

How to prioritize self-care and your mental health. (n.d.). Nivati. https://www.nivati.com/blog/how-to-prioritize-self-care-and-your-mental-health

Hwang, K. O. (2020). Type 2 diabetes: A doctor's guide to a good appointment. *Healthline Media*. https://www.healthline.com/health/type-2-diabetes/guide-to-appointment#What-to-share-with-your-doctor

Importance of medication adherence in diabetes. (2018). Apollo Sugar Clinics. https://apollosugar.com/world-of-diabetes/diabetes-management/importance-of-medication-adherence-in-diabetes/

Injury-free exercise tips. (n.d.). ADA. https://diabetes.org/healthy-living/fitness/getting-started-safely/injury-free-exercise-11-quick-safety-tips

Inspirational stories. (2019). Know Diabetes by Heart. https://www.knowdiabetesbyheart.org/resources/inspiring-stories/

Insulin. (n.d.). Cleveland Clinic. https://my.clevelandclinic.org/health/articles/22601-insulin

Insulin resistance. (n.d.). WebMD. https://www.webmd.com/diabetes/insulin-resistance-syndrome

1 in 10 people are living with diabetes. International Diabetes Federation (IDF) https://www.idf.org/52-about-diabetes/43-rights-and-responsibilities.html

Is diabetes a disability? Understanding your rights and benefits. (2023). Disability Works, https://disabilityworks.org/is-diabetes-a-disability-understanding-your-rights-and-benefits/

Janaway, D. B. (2017). Understanding diabetes jargon. *Patient.* https://patient.info/news-and-features/understanding-diabetes-jargon

Jaspan, R. (2022). 1-Week meal plan & recipe prep for pre-diabetes. *Verywell Fit.* https://www.verywellfit.com/1-week-pre-diabetic-meal-plan-ideas-recipes-and-prep-6504170

Kalra, S., Jena, B. N., & Yeravdekar, R. (2018). Emotional and psychological needs of people with diabetes. *Indian Journal of Endocrinology and Metabolism, 22*(5). https://doi.org/10.4103/ijem.IJEM_579_17

Lachtrupp, E. (2021). Diabetes meal plan for beginners. *EatingWell.* https://www.eatingwell.com/article/7886108/diabetes-meal-plan-for-beginners/

Lando, H. M., & Ragone, M. (2001). Case study: A 68-year-old man with diabetes and peripheral neuropathy. *Clinical Diabetes, 19*(3), 122–123. https://doi.org/10.2337/diaclin.19.3.122

Landry, J. (2023, February 17). *72+ best diabetes quotes and sayings for inspiration (2023).* Respiratory Therapy Zone. https://www.respiratorytherapyzone.com/diabetes-quotes/

Lee, A. M. I. (2019). Self-Advocacy: What it is and why it's important. *Understood.* https://www.understood.org/en/articles/the-importance-of-self-advocacy

Lee, A. R. (2022). How do insulin and blood sugar work in diabetes? *Verywell Health*. https://www.verywellhealth.com/insulin-vs-blood-sugar-how-to-manage-type-2-diabetes-6740387

Lee, A. R. (2023). Drugs that raise blood sugar and can complicate diabetes. *Verywell Health*. https://www.verywellhealth.com/list-of-drugs-that-raise-blood-sugar-6542910

Leung, E., Wongrakpanich, S., & Munshi, M. N. (2018). Diabetes management in the elderly. *Diabetes Spectrum, 31*(3), 245–253. https://doi.org/10.2337/ds18-0033

Lifestyle changes can prevent or delay diabetes. (2022). Verywell Health. https://www.verywellhealth.com/lifestyle-changes-for-diabetes-prevention-6543350

Lifestyle vs. Medication: Which is More Powerful for Maintaining a Healthy Weight? (2016). Ask The Scientists. https://askthescientists.com/lifestyle-improvements-effective-medications-reducing-diabetes-risk/

Living healthy with diabetes. (2018). Www.Heart.Org. https://www.heart.org/en/health-topics/diabetes/prevention--treatment-of-diabetes/living-healthy-with-diabetes

Living my best life with type 2 diabetes. (2020). WebMD. https://www.webmd.com/diabetes/diabetes-perspectives-21/type-2-everyday-life

Lodhia, H. (2023). The power of self-care: Prioritizing mental health in a busy world! *My Publication*. https://drhenalodhia.substack.com/p/the-power-of-self-care-prioritizing

Managing stress when you have diabetes. (n.d.). WebMD. https://www.webmd.com/diabetes/managing-stress

Marcin, A. (2018). *How are carbohydrates digested?* Healthline Media. https://www.healthline.com/health/carbohydrate-digestion#digestion-process

MBE, D. S. J. (2021). Why type 2 diabetes check-ups are so important. *Patient*. https://patient.info/news-and-features/why-you-should-go-for-regular-check-ups-if-you-have-type-2-diabetes

McCament-Mann, L. A. (n.d.). A New Class of Drugs for Diabetes. *National Capital Poison Center*. https://www.poison.org/articles/benefits-and-risks-new-diabetes-drugs-183

McCoy, K. (). The history of diabetes. *EverydayHealth.Com*. https://www.everydayhealth.com/diabetes/understanding/diabetes-mellitus-through-time.aspx

Meds that can spike your blood sugar. (n.d.). WebMD. https://www.webmd.com/diabetes/medicines-blood-sugar-spike

Meissner, M. (2021). How diabetes affects men vs. women. *Medical News Today.* https://www.medicalnewstoday.com/articles/diabetes-affects-men-women

Metabolic syndrome. (2021). Johns Hopkins Medicine. https://www.hopkinsmedicine.org/health/conditions-and-diseases/metabolic-syndrome

Metabolic syndrome—Symptoms and causes. (2021). Mayo Clinic. https://www.mayoclinic.org/diseases-conditions/metabolic-syndrome/symptoms-causes/syc-20351916

Muccioli, M. (2022). Are people with diabetes immunocompromised? *Diabetes Daily.* https://www.diabetesdaily.com/blog/author/mariamuccioli/

National Diabetes Statistics Report. (2022). CDC. https://www.cdc.gov/diabetes/data/statistics-report/index.html

National DPP Customer Service Center. (n.d.). https://nationaldppcsc.cdc.gov/s/article/CDC-2022-National-Diabetes-Statistics-Report

Nellis, P. (2021). Self-Advocacy leads to better health & well-being. *Occupational Therapy Services.* https://otservices.wustl.edu/self-advocacy-leads-to-better-health-well-being/

New technologies in diabetes care and management. (2023). NIDDK: National Institute of Diabetes and Digestive and Kidney Diseases. https://www.niddk.nih.gov/health-information/professionals/diabetes-discoveries-practice/new-technologies-in-diabetes-care-and-management

Normal fasting and postprandial blood glucose levels. (2018). Diabetestalk.Net. https://diabetestalk.net/blood-sugar/normal-fasting-and-postprandial-blood-glucose-levels

Oral and non-insulin medications. (2016). The Johns Hopkins Patient Guide to Diabetes. https://hopkinsdiabetesinfo.org/treatments/oral-medications/

Osborn, C. O. (2020). Type 1 and type 2 diabetes: What's the difference? *Healthline Media.* https://www.healthline.com/health/difference-between-type-1-and-type-2-diabetes

Pacheco, D. (2020a). Diabetes and sleep: Sleep disturbances & coping. *Sleep Foundation.* https://www.sleepfoundation.org/physical-health/lack-of-sleep-and-diabetes

Pacheco, D. (2020b). Sleep & glucose: How blood sugar can affect rest. *Sleep*

Foundation. https://www.sleepfoundation.org/physical-health/sleep-and-blood-glucose-levels

Pancreas. (n.d.). Cleveland Clinic. https://my.clevelandclinic.org/health/body/21743-pancreas

Panoff, L. (2022, November 28). Obesity and diabetes: Connection, risk, and management. *Verywell Health*. https://www.verywellhealth.com/obesity-and-diabetes-6823190

Patient stories. (). The Johns Hopkins Patient Guide to Diabetes. https://hopkinsdiabetesinfo.org/patient-stories/

Pon, E. du, Wildeboer, A. T., van Dooren, A. A., Bilo, H. J. G., Kleefstra, N., & van Dulmen, S. (2019). Active participation of patients with type 2 diabetes in consultations with their primary care practice nurses—What helps and what hinders: A qualitative study. *BMC Health Services Research*, *19*(1), 1–11. https://doi.org/10.1186/s12913-019-4572-5

Poulson, B. (2021). Type 2 diabetes complications: Overview and more. *Verywell Health*. https://www.verywellhealth.com/type-2-diabetes-complications-5120942

Prevalence of Diagnosed Diabetes. (2022). CDC. https://www.cdc.gov/diabetes/data/statistics-report/diagnosed-diabetes.html

Price, C. (2013). A diabetes exercise success story. *ASweetLife*. https://asweetlife.org/a-diabetes-exercise-success-story/

Purdie, J. (2016). Stress: How it affects diabetes and how to decrease it. *Healthline Media*. https://www.healthline.com/health/diabetes-and-stress

Ries, J. (2020). 40% of people with type 2 diabetes initially avoid insulin therapy. *Healthline Media*. https://www.healthline.com/health-news/why-delaying-insulin-is-dangerous-in-the-long-run

Rowley, W. R., Bezold, C., Arikan, Y., Byrne, E., & Krohe, S. (2017). Diabetes 2030: Insights from yesterday, today, and future trends. *Population Health Management*, *20*(1). https://doi.org/10.1089/pop.2015.0181

Sample menu for patients with diabetes. (n.d.). Sutter Health. https://www.sutterhealth.org/health/diabetes/diabetic-meal-plan

Seery, C. (2019). Diabetes real life stories. *Diabetes*. https://www.diabetes.co.uk/diabetes-real-life-stories.html

Shaikh, J. (2021). Why is diabetes increasing in the United States? MedicineNet. https://www.medicinenet.com/why_is_diabetes_increasing_in_the_united_stat/article.htm=

Singh, K. (2019a). Diabetes jargon, abbreviations, and terminology. *Diabetes.* https://www.diabetes.co.uk/diabetes-jargon.html

Singh, K. (2019b). Poor blood circulation - Causes, association with diabetes, treatment. *Diabetes.* https://www.diabetes.co.uk/diabetes-complications/poor-blood-circulation.html

Smoking and diabetes: What you should know. (n.d.). WebMD. https://www.webmd.com/diabetes/smoking-and-diabetes

Spritzler, F. (2020). How many carbs should you eat if you have diabetes? *Healthline Media.* https://www.healthline.com/nutrition/diabetes-carbs-per-day#daily-intake

Srakocic, S. (2022). Blood sugar level charts for type 1 and type 2 diabetes. *Healthline Media.* https://www.healthline.com/health/diabetes/blood-sugar-level-chart#recommended-ranges

Sherrell, Z. (2022). How do diabetes rates vary by country? *Medical News Today.* https://www.medicalnewstoday.com/articles/diabetes-rates-by-country

Steroids and diabetes: What you need to know. (2022). *Diabetes Daily.* https://www.diabetesdaily.com/learn-about-diabetes/treatment/other-drugs/steroids-and-diabetes-what-you-need-to-know/

Tello, C. (2019). 7 benefits of insulin & 2 negative effects. *SelfHacked.* https://selfhacked.com/blog/insulin-101/

Todd, J., Rudaizky, D., Clarke, P., & Sharpe, L. (2021). Cognitive biases in type 2 diabetes and chronic pan. *The Journal of Pain, 23*(1), 112–122. https://doi.org/10.1016/j.jpain.2021.06.016

The Diabetes Site. (2018, April 17). Diabetes and circulation: How to get the blood flowing again. *The Diabetes Site News.* https://blog.thediabetessite.greatergood.com/diabetes-circulation/

The Elderly and diabetes: Everything you need to know. (2016). TheDiabetesCouncil.Com. https://www.thediabetescouncil.com/the-elderly-and-diabetes-everything-you-need-to-know/

The Healthline Editorial Team. (2014). *How is type 2 diabetes diagnosed? What you need to know.* Healthline Media. https://www.healthline.com/health/type-2-diabetes/diagnosis#symptoms

The importance of exercise when you have diabetes. (2018). Harvard Health. https://www.health.harvard.edu/staying-healthy/the-importance-of-exercise-when-you-have-diabetes

The sweet danger of sugar. (2017). Harvard Health. https://www.health.harvard.edu/heart-health/the-sweet-danger-of-sugar

The unselfish art of prioritizing yourself. (2017). Psychology Today. https://www.psychologytoday.com/us/blog/compassion-matters/201708/the-unselfish-art-prioritizing-yourself

Tips for managing diabetes in the childcare setting. (n.d.). ADA. https://diabetes.org/tools-support/know-your-rights/safe-at-school-state-laws/special-considerations/tips-child-care-setting

Turbert, D. (2021). Diabetic eye disease. *American Academy of Ophthalmology.* https://www.aao.org/eye-health/diseases/diabetic-eye-disease

Type 2 diabetes. (n.d.). Diabetes UK. https://www.diabetes.org.uk/diabetes-the-basics/types-of-diabetes/type-2

Type 2 diabetes—Diagnosis and treatment. (2023). Mayo Clinic. https://www.mayoclinic.org/diseases-conditions/type-2-diabetes/diagnosis-treatment/drc-20351199

Understanding diagnosis and treatment of diabetes. (n.d.). WebMD. https://www.webmd.com/diabetes/news/20210629/best-blood-sugar-meds-for-type-2-diabetes

Vieira, G. (2018). How diabetes raises your risk for all major cancers. *Healthline Media.* https://www.healthline.com/health-news/diabetes-raises-risk-for-major-cancers

Watts, M. (2019). Diabetes and counting calories. *Diabetes.* https://www.diabetes.co.uk/features/diabetes-counting-calories.html

Weekly exercise targets. (n.d.). ADA. https://diabetes.org/healthy-living/fitness/weekly-exercise-targets

Weisenberger, J. (2023). *Lifestyle or Drugs to Control Diabetes? Which is Better?* https://jillweisenberger.com/lifestyle-changes-versus-drugs-diabetes-management/

What are some of the risk factors for type 2 diabetes? (2014). Healthline. https://www.healthline.com/health/type-2-diabetes-age-of-onset#risk-factors-for-adults

What are the most difficult challenges for diabetics? (n.d.). Quora. from https://www.quora.com/What-are-the-problems-faced-by-diabetes-patients

What can happen if my blood sugar is out of control? (n.d.). WebMD. https://www.webmd.com/diabetes/uncontrolled-blood-sugar-risks

What does a diabetic ulcer look like? (2019). https://www.medicalnewstoday.com/articles/320739

What high blood sugar does to your body. (n.d.). WebMD. https://www.webmd.com/diabetes/how-sugar-affects-diabetes

What is insulin resistance? A Mayo Clinic expert explains. (2022). [Video]. In *Mayo Clinic.* https://www.mayoclinic.org/diseases-conditions/obesity/multimedia/vid-20536756

Why Technology is Integral to Diabetes Care Management. (n.d.). HealthLeaders Media. rom https://www.healthleadersmedia.com/technology/why-technology-integral-diabetes-care-management

Woolley, E. (2012). How insulin works and why you need it. *Verywell Health.* https://www.verywellhealth.com/how-insulin-works-in-the-body-1087716

Woolston, C. (2020). Diabetes: Safety alerts and emergencies. *Consumer Health News | HealthDay.* https://consumer.healthday.com/encyclopedia/diabetes-13/diabetes-management-news-180/diabetes-safety-alerts-and-emergencies-644104.html

Wright, S. A. (2017). Everything you need to know about glucose. *Healthline Media.* https://www.healthline.com/health/glucose#What-is-glucose?

Yetman, D. (2021, June 23). What to know about diabetes and metabolism. *Healthline Media.* https://www.healthline.com/health/diabetes/diabetes-and-metabolism#metabolism-and-diabetes

What does a diabetic ulcer look like? (2019). https://www.medicalnewstoday.com/articles/320739

What high blood sugar does to your body. (n.d.). WebMD. https://www.webmd.com/diabetes/how-sugar-affects-diabetes

What is insulin resistance? A Mayo Clinic expert explains. (2022). [Video]. In *Mayo Clinic.* https://www.mayoclinic.org/diseases-conditions/obesity/multimedia/vid-20536756

Why Technology is Integral to Diabetes Care Management. (n.d.). HealthLeaders Media. rom https://www.healthleadersmedia.com/technology/why-technology-integral-diabetes-care-management

Woolley, E. (2012). How insulin works and why you need it. *Verywell Health.* https://www.verywellhealth.com/how-insulin-works-in-the-body-1087716

Woolston, C. (2020). Diabetes: Safety alerts and emergencies. *Consumer Health News | HealthDay.* https://consumer.healthday.com/encyclopedia/diabetes-13/diabetes-management-news-180/diabetes-safety-alerts-and-emergencies-644104.html

Wright, S. A. (2017). Everything you need to know about glucose. *Healthline Media.* https://www.healthline.com/health/glucose#What-is-glucose?

Yetman, D. (2021, June 23). What to know about diabetes and metabolism. *Healthline Media.* https://www.healthline.com/health/diabetes/diabetes-and-metabolism#metabolism-and-diabetes

www.ingramcontent.com/pod-product-compliance
Lightning Source LLC
Chambersburg PA
CBHW070624030426
42337CB00020B/3907